CORY MARTIN

LOVE SICK

A Memoir

WRITE OUT PUBLISHING
CALIFORNIA

Published by Write Out Publishing

Published in the United States by
Write Out Publishing, California
www.writeoutpublishing.com

Some names have been changed to protect the privacy of the individuals involved.

Jacket photo: Nicolaes van Verendael
A swag of roses, peonies, anemones, snowballs, carnations, and other flowers hanging from ribbons before a stone niche, with butterflies, caterpillars and other insects, c. 1680
Interior design by Susan Leonard

Library of Congress Control Number: 2015916743

ISBN 978-0-9969193-0-2 hardcover
ISBN 978-0-9969193-1-9 ebook

Printed in the United States of America

1 3 5 7 9 10 8 6 4 2

First Edition

To anyone who's ever felt unlovable;
forget that, you're lovable.

Love Sick

Part 1

Chapter One

FLYING HIGH

I am on drugs. Fucked up, wandering aimlessly, staring at the white haze around me.

I am 28 years old. It is 11 in the morning. I should be sober.

No respectful adult gets high on a Tuesday unless they're famous. I am not famous.

I have taken one and a half pills of Valium. All five feet and four inches of my yoga-toned body feels out of place. I am wearing nothing but a blue hospital gown, a pair of panties and my Nikes.

My neurologist prescribed the pills to ease my nerves, but the people around me don't know I have taken the drugs. This fact makes me jittery, jumpy. Everything feels heightened, like I can hold the oxygen in the room by simply cupping my hands as if it's water to be splashed upon my face. I grasp the air and press it against my sun-kissed skin and laugh. I am loopy, giddy. I attempt restraint. I am hyperaware of my surroundings. I wonder what others think of me. I don't want them to think I'm a degenerate; that getting messed up is something I do regularly. I turn my head. A toddler's logic of hide and seek, if I can't see you then you can't see me. There are two other people in the room. I want them to know that I am smart and intelligent, not a blonde idiot bumbling her way through life, high on looks and Valium.

I focus on the ground.

I prepare a sentence in my head. Over and over to get it right. *Should. I. Go. Here.* Then it drips from my lips.

"Should I go here?" I gesture to the cold bed of an MRI machine.

The technician nods and I hoist myself onto the plasticized gurney. He covers me with a white blanket. A red laser light beams down on my skull to determine the correct placement of the scans about to occur. A soft breeze comes out of the tunnel behind me. A bolster is placed under my knees for comfort. The man gently locks my head in place with a plastic brace then pushes a button to move the bed into the machine. Inside the shaft of the mega magnet he instructs me not to move.

I lie still, but my mind keeps going.

Outside the door, the technician talks to his colleague. They whisper their thoughts to each other. I am certain they are looking at my file. I wonder if they feel sorry for me. I know what it says. I know what they are looking for. I close my eyes. I want to think of pretty things, bright things. I practice inhaling and exhaling through my nose, a technique I have learned to calm myself.

The MRI roars to life. Screaking out sound. Beep. Beep. BEEEEP. The high-pitched note pounds at my ears, a reminder that I am here, doing this right now.

I wonder how much a flight to Maui would cost if I left tomorrow. The last time I was there I was a freshman in college and learned to surf. Maybe I can go shopping after this and buy a new bikini.

"You okay?" the technician asks over the intercom system.

I say yes, then wonder if he can see what I am thinking.

My brain is doing the thing it does when it's decided it no longer wants to be in a place. Jumping from thought to thought. Pulling up memories in a non-sequitur fashion. The first time I crashed a bike. Middle school band. Walking on hot coals with Tony Robbins.

In 1990 my parents bought earthquake insurance. Iben Browning had predicted there would be an event on the New Madrid Fault. The fault spanned from Missouri to Indiana to Illinois, Ohio, and Kentucky. Our house was in the northwest corner of Indiana. Instead of regular tornado drills in school we now had earthquake drills.

"Are you still doing alright?" the technician asks. His voice reverberates through the tube like the wizard from Oz. The machine is mic'd, but I cannot see a soul.

He is looking for something specific on my brain. Reasons for a year-long cycle of pain in my body, numbness that comes and goes but stays longer than it's away. Memory loss, confusion of words, and other symptoms that I've been ignoring for far too long.

I take a deep breath.

My body trembles from the weight of the magnets moving around me. I feel like a fiend, edgy and shaky. I speculate how long Valium stays in the body. One hour? Two?

My ex-boyfriend is picking me up when this is over. He and I once lived together. We cohabitated out of love and convenience. I was only 23. We broke up after six months. He lived with me for two more.

I close my eyes against the white monotony around me. The MRI pounds through its second cycle. My thoughts continue hopping—one foot, then two, a game of hopscotch to ten.

My mom's propensity for preparation is unbelievable. When the Y2K hit, our bathtubs were full of water, the basement had rations of canned food, batteries, giant candles, and more water.

I was home from college in Los Angeles that winter of 1999 and spent the New Year sipping champagne with my parents and sister on the southern shore of Lake Michigan. I was not allowed to celebrate with my friends in Chicago, a city whose lights I could see across the great lake. My mom was paranoid she'd lose us. If the world ended, we'd leave it together.

I have been in three earthquakes since I moved to California at the age of 18. Right now I am in Santa Monica lying in a medical facility 24 blocks from the Pacific Ocean. In my closet at home there is a 40-pound survival kit sent to me by my mom. Should I need them, there are two more pills in my purse prescribed by my doctor.

"We've got about 30 minutes to go," the technician says. "You still doing okay?"

I answer yes. The brain-scanning machine continues its work, vibrating with noise. Buzzing. Buzzing. Its sound crescendos. The soft foam of a set of earplugs protects my eardrums, preventing any ringing that would echo the sounds of this experience for hours to come.

The first earthquake I ever felt struck in the middle of the night. It was the summer between my sophomore and junior years of college. I was living in an apartment just off campus. My twin bed was against one wall. My surfboard was against the other. The board slid down the wall and crashed onto the floor. I hid under my covers. It was not the response I was taught in middle school.

Several months before I found myself here, I moved out of a rent-controlled apartment in Santa Monica to a place in Marina Del Rey, just south along the LA coast. My apartment now looks east out onto the harbor. If a tsunami hits, the water would rush through my neighbor's and straight through my front door.

The MRI becomes silent. Images of my brain are uploaded to a radiologist in a dark room.

The technician re-enters the room and the bed I am on begins to move. "We have one more scan to do," he starts, "but your doctor requested this be done with contrast."

I stare at him blankly.

"I'm going to inject some dye into your arm, wait about a minute, then I'll move you back inside."

"Fine," I say.

The technician shoots the dye into the biggest vein of my right arm as if it were heroin. I feel tingly all over. My nose starts to itch. I reach for it, but I am directed once again to remain still.

"Are you ready?" the technician asks.

I mutter yes, then think about the fact that my insurance will pay for most of this MRI, but the rest I will have to settle with my savings.

The machine comes to life one last time, working itself into a pattern of Morse code. Dash. Dot. Dash. Dot. Pound. Pound. Pound.

I concentrate on the sounds around me, the vibrations move through my body. I read once that monks use the resonance of their voices to heal people. Or was it a shaman?

Or a drum? Images of indigenous tribes spring to mind. Women and elders caring for the sick. It's a tableau of health and yet I'm back to fourth grade glancing over the boys' shoulders at the National Geographic they hold, giggling at the site of real life boobies. I wonder if those women ever get mammograms. The MRI pounds harder.

After ten minutes the room is silent.

"You're all done," the technician says.

I open my eyes. The light in the tube is an ambient yellow. The electronic bed conveys my body past the red laser and into the open air. The cage is unlocked from my skull. I am still a little high.

I sit up and turn to the man. I practice the sentence in my head: *What. Did. You. See.* Then it seeps from my lips.

"When will I get the results?"

"Your doctor should call you in a couple days," he says, then smiles with an apathetic turn of his lips.

I try to read his face for clues, but there is nothing. I exit the metal free zone of the imaging center.

In a small curtained area in the ladies room I redress myself. In the mirror I catch a glimpse of my light green eyes staring back at me. My highlighted blonde hair falls past my shoulders. I grasp for air and place my hands on my cheeks.

The first time I got high was in the basement of my friend Matt's house. I was 16. He was two years older than me and incredibly smart, the kind of guy all moms want their daughters to date. Today he is a doctor in Kentucky.

At the end of this week I will see my doctor.

I gather my things and leave. Outside I wait for my ride on the corner of Wilshire and 24th. A Whole Foods market sits across the way. My purse rattles with the remaining Valium as I shift my weight from side to side. I contemplate taking one more pill, but decide against it. My ex picks me up minutes later and I buy him a slice of pizza as a thank you for acting as my chauffeur. I say little about the exam and crack jokes using what high I have left to forget about the experience.

After he drops me off at my place, I sit on the patio of my apartment and watch as the setting sun's light reflects off the water of the marina. Kids play at the beach below as I come down from my buzz. I think about the day's events then make a mental note of the contents of the emergency kit in my closet. Inside are rations of water, a blanket, some M&Ms, a pile of MREs, toilet paper, and plastic gloves.

Chapter Two

PRETTY WOMAN

"**Y**ou don't get to eat my pussy for free!" screamed out the prostitute as she finished servicing my sex-starved neighbor.

Let me explain…

I believe in moments. Big moments, actually. The kinds of moments that you look back on later in life, point to, and say, "That's when it all changed."

I like to theorize and hypothesize about why my life is the way it is today, and I believe those feline-inspired words at the top of this page are the reason I am where I am right now.

My neighbor, who I'd nicknamed "Mr. Hacker" for his loud smoker's cough that barked up phlegm and a congestion of noise on a nightly basis, had ordered a call girl that May evening of 2007. It was just about midnight on a Tuesday when I heard the moans of a climactic orgasm followed by a request for cash. A request that was, apparently, denied.

Now, I see nothing wrong with a man in his sixties who weighs all of about one hundred pounds and looks like Timothy McVeigh ordering in a little vagina. But when he refused to pay the bill, and she threatened to call her husband to come and shoot him, then made mock shotgun noises, and he threw her against the wall, I drew the line and called the police.

I called 911 and explained the situation. I left out the part about what my neighbor didn't get to do for free and told them there was a prostitute next door and she and Mr. Hacker were now throwing each other against the wall. From the sounds of it she most likely had a gun, and considering the fact that my slumlord apartment had walls like cardboard, I was quite certain that if someone shot, the bullet would blaze right through Mr. Hacker's bedroom wall and straight into mine.

This kind of mayhem was not what you'd expect in a Santa Monica neighborhood on Fourth Street just north of Wilshire, where two-bedroom condos went for $800,000. No, this was the kind of thing that was supposed to happen down on Crenshaw in Compton or Watts.

I hid in my kitchen and cracked the sliding glass door open so that when the police finally arrived I could hear everything. Of course, no one wanted to admit what (or who) was going down minutes prior and the pretty woman and the hacker apologized for the disturbance, telling the cops they got into a "little fight."

When I heard the word *little,* I wondered if that was the loose woman's way of getting back at Mr. Hacker. I pictured her telling the cop, "It was just a small fight," as she held up her pinky finger to indicate that hacker man's penis was "only a slight disturbance."

The image produced only one thought in my mind.

I had to move.

I'd been living in my fabulously rent-controlled one-bedroom apartment since I was 22, and I was going to turn 28 that August. I loved my place and didn't want to leave, but I could see this night for what it was. The hooker and the hacker signified the end of an era and the beginning of something new. This night was one of those life moments that drives you down a different path.

I spent the next few days looking for a new apartment. I started in Santa Monica and headed south along the Los Angeles coast, stopping at every building that had security along the way. Finally, I found my dream apartment. A big complex in Marina Del Rey. It had a pool, a Jacuzzi, tennis courts, a workout room, and everything was gated. Sure, it cost more, but the way I looked at it, if someone could afford the rent there, then they would obviously be able to pay their prostitutes. And that would certainly be a step in the right direction.

On June 6, 2007, I moved into my new apartment with views of the marina and was so ecstatic that I couldn't help beaming from ear to ear. Even though I had lived alone since I was a young 20-something, I finally felt like an adult. This was my first "grown-up" apartment and there was some sixth sense that kept telling me, things were about to change in a major way.

The following week my mom flew out from Chicago to visit and was helping me unpack when she turned to me and said, "I have a feeling, Cory. The next time you move, you're going to be moving into a place with your husband."

"Yeah, right," I laughed, knowing that my track record with guys wasn't so great and the last thing on my mind was a white dress and a walk down the aisle. "I doubt it," I finished.

I was still young and wasn't looking to get married. I had bigger and better ideas. I wanted to write the great American novel, live in a house on the beach, spend weeks in Paris flirting with foreign dignitaries, travel the globe, find myself at an ashram in India...

I looked over at my mom who was now unpacking a box of dishes and my face saddened at the domestic image. I knew she thought she'd made my day by making such a heartfelt prediction. But all I could think was, the impending change cannot be a husband. It has to be something more.

Chapter Three

RIDING SOLO

When I am not high I am a loner.

I like to do my own thing on my own terms. I like going out at night and I like not having to answer to anyone. I like being able to pack a bag and head off to Hawaii for a last minute vacation by myself. I like waking up in the morning and running around my apartment naked. I like walking to the beach and watching the sun set alone. This does not, however, make me a total loser. I have friends. But when shit's going down, I tend to sort through it by myself. It's how I ride. Solo.

In fact, one of my favorite things to do is hop in the car and start driving with no destination in mind. One time I ended up at the Santa Barbara Zoo on a Tuesday, hung out with the giraffes for an hour then drove the two hours home. Right now I am on the Pacific Coast Highway, headed north. I don't know where I'll stop, or if I'll stop, but I like the way the road twists and turns along the Southern California coast.

I practice yoga five days a week, but there is something about driving up this ocean road, windows open, music blasting, that has a larger calming effect on my mind than straight meditation. And seeing how I was just high and confined in an MRI machine one day ago, I am taking this moment to relax and reflect.

The first time I took this drive, I was a student at the University of Southern California. A sophomore studying creative writing, I was a ripe 19-year-old with grandiose visions of living the life of a writer. I was in a poetry class under the tutelage of David St. John. His poetry was magnificent, mine reeked of teenage angst. I was determined to push past that.

On the Saturdays before our weekly poems were due, I would drive up to Malibu in the Volvo sedan my parents had driven out from Indiana. It had once been my father's car. He traveled everywhere in it for work and put 100,000 miles on it within two years. Usually, he would trade his cars in. This one he brought to me. He was a traveling salesman of sorts, but it was good work, the kind of work that paid for me to go to a private school in a very expensive city clear across the country from where I grew up.

The car was the safest on the market. Its green exterior mirrored the shade of the palm fronds above.

Today I drive a light green Jeep. I bought it on my own. On the visor is a warning that the vehicle has a high flip rate at top speeds. I slow down for a second then hit the gas and fly by several Malibu-appropriate convertibles.

In college, the trip from downtown LA, where campus sat, to the edge of Malibu, where I would find myself on a knit blanket my grandmother had made for my dad when he attended college, took anywhere from 40 to 90 minutes. The trip from my apartment in Marina Del Rey now takes 20 minutes.

I've always made this trek solo.

Back then I had a ritual. I'd drive past all the homes, the Malibu Lumber Yard, and Pepperdine University, to find a spot to pull over. There'd be a sign, usually El Matador, and I would park in front of it.

The walk across the PCH was precarious, perfectly timed.

I would hold my blanket in one arm, a notepad in the other.

I'd climb down rocks or a set of rickety stairs. Then I'd set down the blanket and post my body in the perfect spot.

Pen would hit paper and I would write. Sometimes about the view in front of me: the kelp, the sea lions, the kayaker. Sometimes it'd be more obtuse: the air, a whisper, an electric current.

Afterwards, I'd feel recharged. Ready to take on the writing world. Ready to be a for-real writer.

I was 24 when my first book was published. I played it off like it wasn't a big deal. Like, because it was a novelization of a popular TV show it didn't mean anything. But the truth was I was proud. I did the work. I stayed up late and I wrote. I created stories beyond what the audience had seen on the screen and I put thoughts in the characters' heads.

For two years I sustained the momentum as a professional writer. I went from being a producer's assistant, to writing three of those novelizations, to writing two episodes of that once-known TV show *The O.C.* But then the momentum waned and the thoughts I had had on that rock in Malibu, the thoughts that saw the future of me as a writer petered to nothing.

My verbal contract with the executive producers said that I would write one more episode of *The O.C.* that year, and one episode of the spin-off that was in the works.

But the spinoff never happened and I was deemed too young and inexperienced to continue on with *The O.C.*

I didn't have the confidence to sit in the writers' room and pitch stories like all the others. I could write, but I couldn't spout stories on cue. My ideas came to me alone on a rock. They did not easily flow from my mouth.

This had been a truth of mine since I was a young girl. My kindergarten report card says it: *Cory is smart, but very quiet, apprehensive, more of an observer.*

Speaking in front of others did and still does give me hives. Red welts swell on my neck, and engorge with every word I speak. This is not the reaction Hollywood wants you to have to their institution.

So I was let go.

At 26, I was unemployed.

I wrote, but I was wounded. I felt lesser because the words in my head flowed easily onto paper but not from my tongue. My agents sought out other jobs for me. I interviewed, but again I was green, too young.

So I sat at home alone all day, wallowing in the self-pity of my unemployment.

As a way to boost my spirits my dad told me Starbucks would probably hire, plus, he added, they provided insurance. I argued that I already had insurance. For free. From the Writer's Guild of America. Also, TV paid well and I had saved enough money to live an entire year without working. I told him I was an idea person, not a Frappuccino maker.

But he was right and when the money I had saved started to dwindle I went out and found a job that could sustain me.

I work for a husband-and-wife writing team. They write big blockbuster movies. Their films make millions. They respect my opinions. They like my ideas. I research and write and proofread and read everything that comes across their desk. They email work to me and I respond in kind.

There are no meetings. No asking of me to speak in front of others.

It is the perfect situation.

I work from home, I do as I please. I am living the life I want.

But now I am in my Jeep driving north with no direction. My work for the day is done and I am left with my thoughts.

When I was little I pictured myself growing up and moving far from the Midwest, exploring the world city by city. LA to start. A stop in NYC. A few months in the Caribbean, then a hop across the pond.

But no one ever told me how cold a summer in England could be. I learned this firsthand during the months between my junior and senior years of college. I studied abroad at Cambridge University, reading works of fiction written during World War I and World War II and comparing the lives and writings of D. H. Lawrence and Virginia Woolf. I lived above a magic shop and a wine store. The River Cam flowed just beyond where I slept each night. After class each day, I enjoyed pints with friends or took the 45-minute walk out to the Orchard tea garden, where the great writers who had once studied at Cambridge were known to have gathered frequently to share ideas. I fantasized about their lives. I wished I could go back in time and live the way they did: drinking wine, spouting prose, reading at all hours of the night, being part of a circle of artists. It was a romanticized version of the writer's life. One that may have been rife with struggle but one that was full of experience and comrades who understood the way your mind flowed.

To this day, I still contemplate moving there. But the someday, one day, has always remained in the future. There has never been a today. And sometimes I wonder why. Do I not have enough guts? Am I not strong enough to pick up and leave? Could I not figure out how to start a new life? I've done it before. I left Indiana to move to California. I had no friends then. I made a whole new life in LA. I found a way to succeed. But I convince myself that that was different. That I had moved for school, not on a whim. That college had a structure for this type of life change. If I went today, what would I have except an idyllic notion in my head that life on the other side of the pond would be more conducive to the stories in my head?

In college, I had another writing professor who would place a chair in the middle of the room at every class. He called it the obligatory empty chair. We would then be instructed to form a circle around it with our desks as we reviewed each other's short stories. Back then I thought this was my professor's way of expressing his creativity, living up to the idea that all writers were eccentric.

But now I am alone on this road and I know what he was trying to do. He was trying to tell us, more like warn us, that despite the fact that we might be encircled by one or two or tens or hundreds of others, we are like that empty chair, alone in the middle of the room as others create stories around us.

I pull my car over. I am now at the far side of Malibu. There is a seafood joint ahead on the right. Motorcycles fill its parking lot. Tough men and women in leather munch on fish and chips, washing them down with cold beer. I walk across the freeway and stop in a spot above the ocean. I look out across the unending grey blue mass of water. In three days I will get the results of my MRI. If I jumped into the ocean now, I would have to swim around the entire world to make it to England. So instead I stand here in LA looking west, waiting for the tide to come in.

Chapter Four

BIOLOGICAL CLOCK

"**I** CAN'T DO THIS!" I wail into the phone as my dad listens patiently on the other end.

My eyes well up and overflow onto my cheeks. I am sitting in my Marina Del Rey apartment. Outside, couples hold hands as they walk to the beach. Inside, my only company is my purple and red betta fish.

It is Tuesday, October 16, 2007. Exactly four days before my friend Brooke walks down the aisle, and exactly four days before I am to be yet another bridesmaid.

Cars roar by on the street below me. Out my window I watch as the Southern California sun beats down on the water of the marina. Its bright reflection mocks my dark state. The shiny white yachts of the rich and famous of Los Angeles stare back at me as they sway with the incoming tide and I can feel the tears burning at my eyes.

I look at the black bridesmaid dress hanging on the back of my bedroom door. The J. Crew frock is a reminder that I am not the one getting married. And all I can think is, *WHY ME?!*

My dad tries to help. "It's okay. It's okay," he repeats over and over, a mantra to try and calm me. But there is no calming me at this moment.

"Dad!" I gasp into the phone as my lungs seem to collapse beneath the weight of my tears and I curl up into the fetal position on the floor and pound on the sun-bleached carpet of my living room. My white Crate and Barrel couch vibrates with my pain. If it weren't a weekday, I'm certain my neighbors would be calling the cops at the ruckus coming from my apartment.

"What am I going to do?" I cry harder.

"We're gonna get through this," my dad replies. In the background, I can hear my mom asking if it's me again. I've already called them once this morning, just an hour ago. I was upset then too, but now? Now I am far worse.

I'm supposed to be working. Researching the next big Hollywood movie for my A-list-writer bosses, or penning my own blockbuster. Instead, all I can think about is, *How will I do this alone?*

When I woke up this morning, I was just a girl living out her dreams in Los Angeles. I was Ms. Cory Elizabeth Martin (I say Ms. because I think the *M* and the *S* are prettier and more sophisticated at this age than the *M-I-S-S*). I was happy and content and working on my career as a writer. I had figured out how to work from home and still be able to afford a So-Cal lifestyle. I was no longer the insecure young 20-something I had been just a few years ago. I was a confident, strong woman.

"I want my mommy," I whimper, as I continue to clutch at the carpet with my newly manicured nails.

"She's here. We're both here," my dad says. My mom picks up the other line.

"Cory," she says, "It's going to be okay. I promise."

"But what if? What if?" I ask. "What if it's not? What if she's right?"

"We'll take it one step at a time."

And that's when I hear the neurologist's words in my head. Just as clear as they were a few hours ago, right before I left her office.

I believe you have multiple sclerosis.

"But I don't want to be SICK!" I scream.

That morning I had had a follow-up appointment to the MRI of my brain. The MRI showed five lesions, and because my vitamin B12 levels were normal, and I didn't have Lyme disease, cancer, lupus, rheumatoid arthritis, a brain tumor, diabetes, or thyroid problems, the doctor had no other explanation for the lesions and the random numbness and pins and needles sensations I was experiencing in my limbs on a daily basis, except for MS.

"Mom, I need you!" My body trembles with the weight of reality. I want to reach inside the phone and grab her hand, let my dad hold me as I cry, but I can't.

I can only pull at the rough fibers of the carpet as the neurologist's bomb continues to go off in my head.

Multiple sclerosis.

It just keeps echoing in there, bouncing off every inch of my brain. My diseased brain. The brain that has five spots on it. The spots that serve as five pieces of evidence that something is wrong with my body and one day it will all fail me.

My fingers clench harder and my body continues to curl into a ball. So tight I could almost return to my mother's womb.

"Cory, are you there?" they both ask.

I allow my sobs to get louder, an indication that yes I am still there. The din of the lunch-time traffic adds to the cacophony of my tears. I am only one note in the arrangement of the world's symphony, but I feel like a fallen bass drum. Loud and heavy.

"You can do this. We'll help you. We can fly out there right now."

"Would you?" I ask. I know they would. And this makes me stop crying for a moment. The thought of having my parents right here, right now is the most comforting thing I've ever heard. But then my brain skips like a vinyl record and I go back to this weekend. And the wedding and the fact that the DJ's going to call all the single women to the dance floor where the lovelorn will line up to fight each other over the bouquet, and I'll be one of the oldest out there, and... oh God...

"Who's going to want to marry me now?" I wail into the phone.

"What are you talking about?" my dad responds. "Calm down. This has nothing to do with marriage."

I pause for a second and think. He's right, it doesn't. I've never worried about the who or the when of marriage. I always believed in fate. If it was meant to be, it would be. But now, today, I *am* worried, and I don't know why. I ponder this as another tear drips down my cheek. Then it occurs to me. The reason why I am suddenly scared to be single.

Those spots on my brain don't just indicate disease.

There is a far better scientific explanation.

One of those damn lesions is sitting on my biological clock. And it has made the whole thing explode and go into hyper overdrive. Suddenly I could care less about a successful career, now I want a husband and a family. My mind races in circles, contemplating the *what-ifs,* and *what-nows. Who will marry me now? Can I still have babies? When will I have those kids? Who will love me forever? Who will take me in his arms and hold me tight?*

"Do you want to come home?" my mom asks and I want to scream.

Yes! Yes! Absolutely yes! What better way to pull the plug on that ticking clock than moving back in with your parents? Maybe I could just pack up and leave right now. No good-byes. No explanation. It would be so perfect. And relaxing. So easy to forget… to not have to think about anything… to have no worries… no commitments… no responsibilities… but…

"What about Brooke's wedding?" I wonder aloud. "I can't do that to her."

"I'm sure she'd understand," my dad says calmly.

I'm sure she would, but…

"I think you should go," my mom says with such a "mom authority" that I know she's right. "It'll be good for you to get out and have fun with your friends. Think of it as a mini-vacation. Try not to think about what Dr. Comer said. You'll see a specialist and we'll get more answers then."

The idea of not having to think about the MS for the weekend sounds just like what the doctor ordered. And it's true, the neurologist only said she believed it was MS, perhaps the specialist will have better news and she'll tell me it's not MS at all.

"Okay, I'm going to go," I state with certainty as I gather strength and start to peel myself from the floor.

"That's my girl," my dad says, as if he can see me from three thousand miles away.

"You know you can call us anytime," Mom adds.

"I know," I say as I sit up straight.

"We're going to get through this. We love you," they say in chorus.

"Love you too," I say as I hang up the phone and head to my room.

In the corner of my bedroom there is a cubby-hole office. It's a large white Pottery Barn desk with a bookshelf on the back of it. My first instinct is to sit at the computer and record my thoughts, sort through this madness that I am now experiencing, but when I walk into my room and nearly trip over my empty suitcase, I find a new resolve.

I take a turn before I reach my desk and fling open the doors to my closet. I push back the hangers and find the sexiest dress I own to wear to the rehearsal dinner and two pairs of the laciest thongs I've ever seen. After all, aren't weddings supposed to be the perfect place to meet someone? Maybe I'll get lucky and catch the bouquet.

Chapter Five

MAN HANDS

I have man hands. I am telling you this because: A) I am a girl and it's the equivalent of me saying how fat I am with the hopes that you'll respond, "You're not fat." And B) You may be the man I marry one day and you should know. I need a big ring. And when I say big, I do not mean one carat. I am talking at least two or more. Designer names are not important but Tiffany is always a great place to start.

I am not telling you this because I am vain, or just out to meet a rich man who can buy me all the bling in the world. I am saying this because it is the truth. My fingers are fat. Plus-size to be exact. If you put a one-carat diamond ring on my hand it will look like a quarter of a carat, and that would be disappointing. Disappointing to you. Disappointing to me. So, I figure I should just save everyone the trouble, heartache, and disappointment and lay all my cards out there on the table. Now you know. My fingers are big and they require even bigger rings to mask their size. Some girls wear black and a pair of Spanx, I don chunky rings.

The reason I bring all of this up is because there is a story I think you need to hear. About the day I thought my giant-ring-wearing days were over.

Christmas time, 2004. Three years before I had ever set foot in a neurologist's office.

I had just finished work for the day at my job in Manhattan Beach and was headed south, out of LA to Newport Beach. With the holidays looming around the corner and writing on the television show I had been working on slowing down, I was free to enjoy the California winter. I hopped in my little Jeep Liberty and weaved through four lanes of traffic on the 405. I was on my way to join friends on their boat as they drove around the harbor in the Christmas Parade. Newport Beach hosts this week-long event every year. And every year, people with giant yachts decorate them with lights and blow-up Santas and drive them around the waterways, drinking Dom Pérignon and bundling up in Burberry scarves. The haute couture lifestyle of Orange County was no shock to me by that point in my life. True, I am just a Midwestern girl from a small Indiana town, who used to think playing hide and seek with the crop dusters in the cornfields behind her yard was the best game ever. But, I had also spent four years at USC, a college whose campus was mainly populated by the spoiled children of the OC, and I was quite familiar with the fact that most kids in the area grew up with BMW-laced birthdays, not cyanide-filled skies. More recently, several of my post-college friends had made the move from Los Angeles down to the Southern California coastal town and I knew the place well.

Emily, one of my good friends, had settled in to the ritzy town to be with her now husband. (As a side note, you should know that her ring is about two and a half carats and she has fairly dainty hands. Not that I would even begin to compare myself to her. But in the interest of full disclosure, I thought you should know.)

I was on my way to meet up with Emily when the intermittent numbness that I had been experiencing and ignoring for several months suddenly struck my left ring finger and rendered it completely useless.

As I bumped and honked and dodged the LA traffic, I tried not to panic, but too many thoughts kept running through my head. *Okay, this is serious. This isn't something you can blame on stress, or a weird sleeping position. This was honest to goodness numbness. Not the kind of numbness you might get in your ass and legs if you sat on the toilet too long. No, this was real. And not going away.*

I started to have a panic attack. My breathing got shallow and I yawned to try and let in a big gulp of air, only to feel my entire throat close up and shut out the outside world. Thanks to trying to write a 300-page book and work a 14-hour-a-day job simultaneously nine months prior to this moment, I easily slipped into panic attack mode whenever I felt an ounce of stress.

The first time it happened I was at work. My producer boss at the time was in a big meeting with some studio head as I sat in a trailer on the Warner Brothers lot in Burbank, fielding phone calls and writing *The O.C.* novelizations. I thought I could drive myself to the ER, but when one of my co-workers asked me where I was going, he insisted on driving.

I was certain I was having an asthma attack and I'd soon be fine, but when the ER doctor walked in and asked me about my recent stress levels, I wondered, *What does my lack of breath have to do with the patch of grey sprouting next to my side part?* But before I could ask, the doctor explained that I had had a panic attack and suggested I look into seeing a therapist. He gave me a handout that explained the physical manifestations of anxiety and stress and sent me on my way. I quickly tossed the evidence of said panic attack into the trash and told the other assistant we better get back to the studio lot before we got fired. Therapy was for the weak and I was strong. So strong that I marched right back to that trailer and worked until eight that night, explaining to my boss that I had had a small asthma attack, but I was fine. Shaun Cassidy, the one-time teenage heartthrob, who was now a TV producer and working on our show, said something about his kid's allergies and the next day my boss sent one of the production peons out to buy a state-of-the art air cleaner from Sharper Image. In true Hollywood fashion, I'd lied and benefited, but at least I didn't have to admit my weakness and I was breathing cleaner air than George Clooney, whose office was just around the corner.

But now, as I sat in traffic, there were no air filters or lies to wash away my panic, and I couldn't help but try to contort my face and neck in any way possible just to feel like there was air in my lungs. The air that was letting me breathe. Survive. Drive to Newport. Not crash. Grow old. Laugh. Live. Shit, where is that air?

Calm down, I tried to tell myself. *It will go away. It always does. This is nothing. You just have some weird circulation issues.*

But when I looked down and saw that my finger wasn't responding to anything, I really freaked. Only, I didn't go into freak-about-my-health mode, instead I went into shallow-girl mode. And I thought...

Your finger's going to die. Rot. Fall off. And then you'll have nothing to put a three-carat diamond on.

Images of some handsome man proposing to me flashed through my head like a fashion photographer on speed.

Click. He's on one knee.

Click. The tears run down my face as he tells me how much he loves me.

Click. He pulls out a small box.

Click. He says the four words. "Will you marry me?"

Click. He reaches for my hand.

Click. My hand is missing a finger.

Click. He pulls away the ring.

Click. The fairy tale is over.

Click…

B-E-E-P! H-O-O-O-N-K!… reality sets back in.

I swerved to avoid a black Range Rover as the *O.C. Chrismukkah* album blared in the background. Jimmy Eat World's "Last Christmas" was on, mocking me. *Last Christmas, I gave you my heart, but the very next day, you gave it away.*

I focused on the road ahead. I wasn't about to give anything away, especially not my finger. I shook my hand again. Maybe I had cut off circulation. Nothing. I massaged it. Nothing. I rubbed it harder. Nothing. *Crap,* I thought. *This is scary.* But at 25, I wasn't thinking that I could possibly have some sort of disease that I would have to live with the rest of my life. All I could think was who's going to give me Cartier if I don't even have a ring finger? Instead, I realized I'd have to wear some Mafioso-esque pinky ring or put it on a chain around my neck, like Carrie Bradshaw did when she realized she wasn't quite ready to marry Aidan.

I tapped my finger on the steering wheel once more, just to see if I could bring back any feeling, but nothing happened. My finger remained useless. The panic began to return. I opened my mouth to breathe. *Please,* I prayed, *I need this air.* My finger was numb and I was about to stop breathing. But to my surprise, I managed to sigh a deep sigh. The air moved through me and a wave of relief washed away the immediate tension. In that moment of bliss, I stepped on the gas and resigned myself to finish my drive down to Newport and do what any good girl with some success at a young age does. Ignore the problem, drink several glasses of wine, and flirt with older men.

For all I knew I was going to wake up the next morning and have to get my ring finger amputated. If I was going down, I was going to go down big. And I was going to find some rich OC man to whisk me away to Vegas, buy me Harry Winston's finest, marry me that night, then divorce me in the morning.

Of course, there was no marriage or a sparkly consolation prize for the annulment, but a few days later, the numbness did finally go away. And for the next three years, I tried to forget that it ever happened. But what I didn't realize was that night was just the beginning of this journey, and over time that numbness began to spread.

First, it was in my hands. Then my arms at night. Then my neck, and my legs as I slept. I blamed it on bad pillows, a cheap bed, lack of exercise, sleeping wrong, but sometimes it turned into a never-ending case of pins and needles. Then, I blamed it on bad food, the moon, pollution. I tried to pretend it wasn't happening, but deep down I knew there was something going on and one day I would have to say something to someone, and that's when fate intervened.

It was May of 2007 when I learned I was about to lose my insurance from the WGA. It was then I realized I had one shot left before the option to get help was gone. I told my regular doctor about the random numbness in my arms, legs, and neck that I had been experiencing and ignoring for the last three years. When I told her I could barely sleep she became concerned and sent me to the neurologist who ran a few blood tests and determined at the time that the cause was most likely a low level of B12. My parents, who had flown to LA for the appointment, immediately bought me a giant bottle of B vitamins and we celebrated that night with a bottle of wine at my favorite Santa Monica restaurant, Giorgio Baldi. We were sure it was nothing serious. I spent the rest of that summer celebrating, thinking I had just dodged a huge bullet. But when fall came around and nothing had improved, I knew that something was seriously wrong.

I had scheduled a follow-up appointment with the neurologist, but I didn't think I could wait for answers, so I got on the internet and started to search for all of my symptoms. On top of the numbness that never went away, I now had trouble remembering the words to finish my sentences, and I couldn't remember the things I'd done just minutes prior. I Googled numbness and memory loss, and in doing so I came across a blog where people discussed their experiences with multiple sclerosis. At the time I knew little about the disease, except I thought everyone who had it was in a wheelchair. Certainly, this couldn't be what I had. I was still walking. But I kept reading anyway and found a post some guy had made that talked about this weird electrical feeling he would get running through his head when he moved his chin towards his chest. Then it hit me.

I had had that same thing. Only I had thought it was the stress of a new job. My first "Hollywood" job, actually. It was September of 2001 and I had been working at a production company as an assistant to the producer. Mainly, I got a lot of coffee. Made sure the fridge was stocked with Tejava tea for the times when Drew Barrymore came by. Listened to Mark McGrath sing "Fly" as he took a shit in our office bathroom and learned to answer phones. I'd been there all of four months when I started getting these weird rolling electrical "headaches" every time I moved my head. I just blew it off and kept on working.

The feelings lasted all through that month. As planes buzzed into the towers of the World Trade Center my head buzzed with the electricity of what I would later discover was my first MS attack.

When I finally returned to the neurologist, she asked me if there were any other incidents I could remember besides the finger thing and all the symptoms I was currently dealing with.

I told her that I believed I had experienced Lhermitte's sign, which was what they called the electrical headaches.

"Is it possible I have MS?" I asked with the hopes that she would tell me not to diagnose myself with things I'd read on the internet, but instead her answer said it all.

"I think we should order an MRI of your brain."

I looked at her with silent tears in my eyes.

Her only response was, "We'll get to the bottom of this." Then she handed me some drug samples to take home. I think she said they were supposed to help with the numbness, so I could finally sleep through the night. To be honest, I wasn't listening. When I got home, I researched the drugs on the internet and discovered that one of the side effects was rapid weight gain, so I decided not to take them.

My fingers were big enough as it was. I didn't need to gain any weight.

Chapter Six

F-U, MS

O MG. FML. I am too old for initial speak, or internet jargon, but this is the kind of shit that's floating around my brain these days.

My life has always been simple, clear cut and easy to understand.

I was born outside of Chicago. Moved to Indiana at the age of ten. Played sports, practiced the piano, made my bed, brushed my teeth, got good grades, went to a fine college, graduated, got a job, paid my bills, lived on my own.

Everything was clearly defined.

But now? Now, in the days after seeing my neurologist? My world is thrown upside down by just two letters and the only definition I have for it all is from the National Multiple Sclerosis Society:

Multiple sclerosis is an immune-mediated process in which an abnormal response of the body's immune system is directed against the central nervous system, i.e., the brain, spinal cord, and optic nerves. When any part of the myelin or nerve is damaged, or destroyed, nerve impulses traveling to and from the brain and spinal cord are distorted or interrupted, producing a wide variety of symptoms.

And all I can think is, *WTF does this all mean for me?*

Multiple sclerosis isn't like cancer or diabetes or HIV. I didn't grow up knowing about it. It wasn't taught in health class and there certainly weren't ads, shows, or movies depicting its effects on someone's life.

It's an enigma. A mysterious force occurring within my body. Only it's not like when I was approaching puberty, and wondering about my growing chest, or that hair down there; it's a whole other beast. No one I know has been through what I'm experiencing. I can't look to older friends, my mom, or aunts, and ask, "What was it like when your arms went numb?"

Instead, it's me at my computer staying up 'til four in the morning researching my future, looking for solace. But comfort is hard to find. There are blogs and websites built around providing information about the disease. Chat rooms filled with horror stories and how to overcome certain factors. The National MS Society has monthly news-letters and quarterly magazines with updates on research and drug trials. And there are plenty of informational sessions at the hospital. But there's nothing to tell me exactly what is going to happen to my body, my life. It's like I've been dealt the broken Magic 8 Ball of diseases. All the answers are clouded and the more I shake things up, the more the bubbles take over.

I'm supposed to be at an age where I feel at home in my own skin, enjoying the prowess of a figure shaped by down dog and the gym, but I can't get behind my own strength. Outwardly I appear strong, inwardly I feel completely disconnected, as if the figure I inhabit is no longer mine. I feel like I'm having some sort of out-of-body experience, only I know this will not lead to any type of spiritual enlightenment no matter how many "oms" I chant. This is a scientific problem, not a metaphysical one. And while I'm no physicist, I know enough to know the equation of my future will not be an easy one to solve.

MS plus X, factor in the variables, divide by Y, take it to the tenth degree and ugh, I'm tired just thinking about it.

But this is my reality, so I keep researching and I discover that I now have to fit into a category. It's like the way my friends and I categorize the men we've dated, only instead of rating things like marriage potential and fuckability, this is a sliding scale of how bad the MS could end up being.

There's the *relapsing-remitting* category of multiple sclerosis, where people have temporary periods called relapses, flare-ups, or exacerbations when symptoms appear.

Then there's the *secondary-progressive* category, where symptoms worsen more steadily over time, with or without relapses.

And then there's *primary-progressive,* where symptoms slowly worsen from the beginning with no relapses or remissions.

And the last category is *progressive-relapsing,* where the disease steadily worsens from the beginning with acute relapses but no remissions, with or without recovery.

Currently I am in the relapsing-remitting category, where my symptoms appear and then disappear, but there's no guarantee that I will stay there.

If more symptoms occur, there's a chance I could recover and then go into remission, but there's also a chance of relapse—and everyone knows when you relapse it just gets harder and harder to break free from the pattern of destruction.

And now I'm wondering, is this what happens with MS? Does it just become a sequence of demolition to the body? Like a pattern of dating the wrong guys, slowly breaking you down until you're a shell of your old existence?

I feel like Oz's Tin Man and Scarecrow and Lion all at once, looking for those one things I think I need. The courage. A heart. A brain.

There is a class of drugs that the FDA has approved to modify the disease, but they scare me. The majority of the ones on the market are injectable, which means I would have to give myself a weekly shot of a drug that could cause pretty severe side effects—all for the possibility of slowing the progression of MS by about 50 percent.

I want to click my heels three times and return home. Instead I click the words "more info" and retrieve more bad news. The wizard of Google is a coward, afraid to tell me my true reality.

It's a sea of vagueness, and I'm starting to drown in it. Instead of working on my writing late at night, I find myself staying up to re-read everything I've already read about the disease. I rehash old thoughts in my mind, and let the constant loop of fear play over and over. I'm afraid to fall asleep, lest one of the symptoms appear overnight. Symptoms like paralysis and blindness. So I stay up late watching medical shows like *Untold Stories of the E.R.* and *Mystery Diagnosis* and I play doctor. I try to figure out what's wrong with the patient before the real MD on the show gives his prognosis.

Night after night, I follow this routine until my couch gains a discernible dip where my body slumbers, passed out from exhaustion. In the mornings I wake up with the sun on my face, but inside I feel like I am living in a room with blackout shades. I check my email to see if my bosses have sent me any work for the day. If they have, I acknowledge it and then I set it aside. I procrastinate with more research on MS, even though I'm probably supposed to be researching story lines for my bosses' next film. Instead, I've created a routine of desperation. My work has slacked and my own writing is nil. I am in what they might call a state of depression, but because I work from home, there's no one to acknowledge it and no one to pull me out of my stupor. Instead, it's me and the internet and the powers of my imagination—creating unpleasant scenarios about my body and the threat of the disease. I am a waste of a human being. Napping, procrastinating, and wallowing in my sorrow. All of this occurs behind closed doors. I keep up enough of an appearance so that no one knows how hard I'm struggling. If you ask my friends, I was a little down and out, but now I'm fine. If you ask me about work, I'm staying up late, pulling all nighters. If you ask, I've got an answer to everything, but it's a giant mirage.

When I was nine I was hired to model in a Hallmark ad. It was for a line of cards called *To Kids with Love*. There's a photo of me in pajamas with a sad face standing above an image of the card that says, "Wish I were there to tuck you in." The card was meant for parents to give to their kids when they were traveling for work. My parents told me not to tell anyone I had done the ad. Extended family members knew, but I was told not to boast. So I stayed quiet and told no one. I suppose it was a good lesson in being humble, unfortunately it's carried over into other aspects of my life and I now have a hard time asking for help or telling people anything about me. The way I see it, no one needs to know about my problems, the same way I shouldn't brag about my accomplishments. It's a convoluted mess I've made in my head, but it's the only way I know. I can talk to my parents and my younger sister Cassie, but to expose myself to others is difficult and a rare occasion. So, I've talked to my friends about what I'm going through, but I've kept it brief and on the surface. Instead of reaching out for help, I stay at home and breakdown on my own. Then I do my best to keep busy with other distractions.

The day after I see the neurologist for my results, I schedule an appointment to get my hair cut and highlighted. I figure that I would make this appointment as a way to cheer myself up. So exactly 53 hours after I contemplated returning home to live with my parents, I am at Fred Segal Salon, sipping white wine while my hairstylist makes small talk. She asks how I am doing and I say I am great. That work and life are going along just fine. I keep the conversation breezy. As I sit under the dryer, the dye brightening my locks, I continue to pretend that life is fabulous. That I can carry on just as I have in the past. Staying quiet and keeping to myself. In some ways it is thrilling. I think of it like some fucked-up kind of weapon. Viewing it as if I could use it as a get-out-of-jail card, if it ever became necessary. I play out various scenarios in my head.

Oh, you want to charge me 75 bucks extra to put a mask on my hair to make it smooth? But I just found out I have MS. Oh, lady with the Botox and jacked up lips: You want to give me a dirty look because I'm not as fake pretty as you are? Well, I just found out I have MS, so I'm not really concerned about superficial things. Oh, meter lady outside: You want to give me a parking ticket? But I just found out I have MS, can't you give me a break?

I did a version of this game as a kid. Any time a boy would make a remark about my appearance, or a girl would put me down, I'd pretend that I didn't care because I had my own secret. In my head I was made famous by Hallmark. I figured one day those kids would see me in a magazine and then they would stop poking fun. But the truth is no one ever knew that my face had appeared on the pages of *People* magazine. The only thing that was real was the fact that their comments hurt. They always did. But I kept up the charade like many kids do and I got through those awkward years. However, MS is not really an awkward phase.

So I keep looking for a way to get back to my simple life. I meditate, I chant. I focus on hippy dippy stuff. Rainbows and daisies and positive thoughts. Then I return to the facts. The science, the medicine, the drug trials, the experiments. Like the honors student I once was, I try to make sense of it all. I make charts. I take notes. I ask questions. But I know that I may never find the answer I want.

Chapter Seven

THE BOUQUET TOSS

I swear I'm not a hoarder. I've never collected chicken carcasses or saved the plastic wrap around my razor blades, but there is a rose I've kept for 15 years. It is the first rose I ever received from a boy who was not my father. In a book filled with mementos, pressed onto a page with a photo of us and a card signed by him, Jason, with the words, "I love you," the red rose is flattened, stained with time and a greying mark of mold. The photo album that holds the preserved flower sits next to tomes gathered over the years. Books from high school, *Great Gatsby,* a Spanish dictionary, books from college, T.C. Boyle, and how-to's on sex, books of life and love, *The Awakening, Our Town,* and poetry and prose, Rumi and Byron and Keats. They're all there on one shelf—a yearbook of my brain, a reminder of the life I've lived. A life I am now contemplating, wondering what's next?

It has been four days since the neurologist told me I most likely have MS and I am in San Diego, alone in a hotel room. My friend Brooke's wedding is this afternoon.

In two hours I will be picked up by another friend who will take me to Brooke's mother's house where I'll be made up to look pretty. My hair and makeup will be professionally done and later I'll stand in line as a witness to the love shared between my friend and her soon-to-be husband.

But now it's seven in the morning and I cannot sleep. I decide I need a distraction from the debilitating thoughts of MS.

I decide I need to swim.

I slip out of my pajamas and cover my girly parts with a black and gold bikini. Adrenaline rushes through me as I walk out to the pool.

As a kid, I was impossible to ply away from the water. My sister and I used to hold auditions for our own *Little Mermaid* productions in the family room. I cast myself as Ariel every time. With one fin covered in sparkly scales, I knew I would forever be beautiful even if I could never walk on land. In high school I swam competitively.

I hop into the hotel pool and start to glide through the water. First freestyle, then breaststroke, then, as the sun gets brighter, I move to butterfly, the hardest of them all.

The muscles of my arms glisten with chlorine. My skin turns a pale brown. Lap after lap, stroke after stroke, I keep swimming. Forty-five minutes straight. When I finally finish, I pause at the side of the pool, my legs dangling in the water, my chin resting on my folded arms atop the deck. Flowers surround the entire area. Yellow hibiscus, and others I cannot name. I breathe in their scent.

I look at my water-logged hands, wrinkled as a small child's. I contemplate nature and its preservation.

Flowers are pretty unless they're dying. But even then you can preserve their beauty, drying them out, or pressing them between the pages of a book.

But what about me?

I press my hands onto the edge of the pool in an exaggerated manner and gracefully pull my body out of the pool in one smooth motion.

Over the next few hours a professional applies makeup to my face to enhance my large lips and bright eyes. Another curls my hair. The other bridesmaids and I sip mimosas as the bride ponders aloud her soon-to-be life as a married woman.

Later, in the garden of the San Diego Museum of Art, I listen to the bride and the groom promise to be there for each other for eternity. I try to pay attention during their vows, but instead I find myself scanning the crowd for the single men. I look for men of stature, who look like they have power; not for the boardroom but for me, for my ailing body.

When I was in college I had this friend, Brian. He liked my roommate, but he would spend almost three nights a week in my bed, cuddling with me. Nothing romantic would ever happen between us. We'd spoon in my extra-long twin bed and hold each other through the night. While I had my friends and my roommate to keep me company most of the time, there was something about the arms of a man that was different. Living clear across the country from my family and all I'd ever known was lonely, and allowing Brian to cocoon my body with his was the one thing that brought me relief.

As my heels sink into the grass, I continue to survey the crowd for loving prospects. I check out each guy and vow to myself that I will not make tonight a night about me and my news. I will make it about moving forward and maybe catching the bouquet.

After the vows are said and the rings exchanged, the party starts and I join in the festivities.

With each song that plays through the speakers, I accept the offer to dance with a new guy. I sample all the goods when it comes to the men and keep my eye on a few. They line up and bring me drinks and sit with me when my feet get tired.

Halfway through the reception the lead singer of the band announces that it is time for the bouquet toss. I see this as my time to shine. I leave my suitors behind, throw my heels to the side and survey my competition. There are girls with longtime boyfriends who've yet to receive a ring, older divorcees, a junior bridesmaid, some pushy relatives, a few other bridesmaids, and me.

I jockey for the best position to catch the flying mass of white and green and the promise of love. A drumroll begins and before I know it the roses float above me. I step left, then right, take two steps back and stretch out my hands but just as I think I have it, the flowers are out of reach.

Someone else has caught the bouquet.

The music stops, the crowd claps, and the photographer takes a photo of the lucky girl and her beautiful smile.

I turn my head. I pick up my shoes and quietly make my way off the dance floor. I can feel tears gathering in the corners of my eyes.

My friends Colleen and Emily see this, grab my hands and lead me to the bathroom. The three of us lock ourselves inside the handicapped stall and I let the tears flow.

"I'm so sorry that you have to go through this," Emily says.

Colleen wraps her arms around me. "Seriously, this sucks."

I hug the girls and they hold me as I cry even harder. This is the first time that the three of us have talked about my diagnosis together in person. I feel their tears drip onto my perfectly coifed hair. Without words we hold each other and acknowledge all our fears. What is going to happen to me? My health? My body? Our friendships? Just days ago we were 20-somethings with so much possibility ahead of us and now we were being shown that life might not be as simple as we'd believed. The thought is out there. If this can happen to me, then what could happen to the rest of us? We are no longer girls who can simply gossip over mani-pedis, sip wine 'til all hours of the night, party like we're still in college, and laugh until we cry.

We are adults now, with real problems and fears and commitments. My struggles have opened the door to a future we know nothing about. We've peeked inside to find that the road ahead is most likely difficult, and if we think harder and look at the world around us, statistics will tell us that there will be marital strife, complicated childbirths, loss of jobs, more sickness, death, financial struggles, moves across the state, the country. I grab my friends' hands and squeeze them tight. I don't want to face this alone.

We look in each others' eyes and make a silent pact to get through this together.

I hug my friends. Then I hear the band playing outside and feel the urge to dance.

Our futures might be uncertain but the one thing we have in this moment is our youth and we can't let our unwrinkled skin go to waste.

"We should get back out there," I say, breaking the silence.

Colleen looks at me then asks, "Are you sure? I can get us more wine from the bar and we can stay in here all night."

"I can get us cake," Emily adds.

I think about it for a moment, and seriously contemplate staying, but then—

"I'm not spending Brooke's wedding in a handicapped stall," I say.

They both agree.

"But, maybe we should fix our makeup," I suggest.

"Yeah," Emily replies. "I saw all those guys you were dancing with."

I smile. There is something about the threat of disease that gives me a false sense of confidence and that confidence has attracted quite a lot of men.

For the rest of the night I continue to dance my way through all of the single boys. When the party starts to dwindle and the buses arrive to take us all to the hotel, I play hard to get with my targets. I board the bus with Colleen and tell the guys that perhaps I'll see them there.

When we arrive at the hotel bar, one shows up at my side immediately. His name is Randy—a perfect Southern California boy at five-foot-ten, with blonde hair and a nice smile. He offers to buy me a drink. I graciously accept.

"I had a lot of fun dancing," he says. "There's something special about you."

"I don't know about that," I reply. But I know there is. It's not special, but it's something, and it's different and it's the reason I will forever be unique when compared to all the other healthy girls around me.

"Well, I think so," he says as he places his warm hand on my forearm.

"Thanks," I reply, unsure of what to say next, except that I like the feeling of his touch, and his skin against mine. "Did you have fun tonight?"

"Yes," he says with a smile and a squeeze to my arm.

We continue to flirt over small talk, and when the lights come on and it's time to go, Randy asks for my number. I, of course, oblige and hand over the ten digits that offer up a direct line to my gold Razr phone.

Two days later, once I return to LA, Randy calls to check in. We make plans for the following Tuesday and when he arrives at my place we take a walk to the Mexican cantina a few blocks from my apartment down by the beach.

I make sure we order margaritas right away as I am having one of those days where my memory and cognition aren't quite the way they used to be, and I am nervous about getting through the basic niceties of the first date.

I let Randy talk first, and as he does, I sip and smile and twirl my hair and keep asking short questions so that he'll have to tell me all about himself while I let the tequila work its magic on my lethargic brain.

Even though I'd thought Randy was at least five years older than me, I quickly discover that he's actually a year younger. He graduated from one of those almost Ivy League schools in the South and was about to finish law school that spring.

I look across the table at my handsome, blue-eyed date in his obligatory prepster uniform of topsiders and a polo shirt and wonder: *What if I do have to use a wheelchair one day? Will Randy leave me or help me get around?* Instead of wondering what he might be like in bed, or what kind of fun trips we might take together, I am caught in a new reality. A dating reality that has me concerned about things no one should ever have to worry about. Like, instead of wondering if he'll be strong enough to open a jar of pickles or pick me up and carry me over the threshold, I am thinking: *Will he be strong enough to fight and protect me if I happen to get stuck in the middle of a shootout or a bank robbery?*

"I applied to the CIA," Randy states in such a matter-of-fact way that I am convinced he knows what I am thinking.

What? I nearly choke on the tequila. "Really?"

"Yeah, right after college," Randy says with a smile and a wink, then tells me how he'd worked two years in diplomatic security before he started law school.

He continues on with details, about how he's already scoped out the restaurant for the quickest exits if he should happen to spot a sniper, but I am back inside my own head. Completely excited. Because, do you want to know the guy that's going to stop the bullets, bring peace to the situation, and carry the disabled girl out the door when she happens to get stuck in a shoot-out?

The man who's been trained by Navy SEALs and Green Berets. That's who.

Hello, Randy. I know we just met, but would you like to marry me?

"Uh, do you want another margarita?" Randy asks. I look down and realize that I have already finished my drink.

"Um, sure, if you're going to have one," I reply, hoping he doesn't think I'm a total lush, but know that if he does it's better than him thinking I have something seriously wrong with me.

We order another drink and I tell him all about myself. There are a few pauses in conversation where I can't remember the words to things or the names of the characters on the TV show I had once written lines for. But all in all, it is a great first date. So great, in fact, that I invite Randy back to my place.

Once inside, I offer him a glass of water and we sit together on my couch. We talk for another hour about our lives. We connect as we converse and soon our words become sparse and our lips meet in the dim light of my apartment. He places his hand on the back of my neck and draws me in closer. I can feel his breath on my forehead and when he kisses the top of my head my body melts. I want him to spend the night, but when he gets up to leave an hour later, at three in the morning, and we are still fully dressed, I know that something is different about him and us.

Chapter Eight

DEMOCRATS FOR CHANGE

I kissed a girl once. Maybe twice. To be honest, I barely remember. It was one of those drunken college things that just sort of happened. The truth is, I'm straight. And kind of conservative (that's what happens when you grow up in the middle of America). But I've lived in California for ten years. So, when it comes to politics, I fall right in the middle. And like my co-ed curiosity for a girl's soft lips, I like to check out each side of the political spectrum. I guess you could say I'm bi-curious, mixing a little of the left with the right.

However, had I known I would one day soon get the news of MS, I might have decided to lean a little further to the left and embraced the political experience in nothing but bra and panties, rather than with just a kiss.

Thursday, March 22, 2007, Elizabeth Edwards stands by her husband's side as she announces to the world that her cancer has come back. It is now in her bones and incurable.

Friday, March 23, 2007, I am in the parking lot of Supermarine at the Santa Monica Airport. If you have never been here, it is where the private planes of the rich and famous land and depart. I am waiting for a certain Hawker

800XP. On that plane are John and Elizabeth Edwards. They are my passengers for the day. No, I am not some sort of limo driver or taxi service, I am just a girl with a few friends in politics who were desperate for a volunteer.

So, now I wait in the black Cadillac that Heather Thomas, yes, the Heather Thomas of *The Fall Guy* fame, has rented for me. I am sitting with John Davis, who is Senator Edwards's go-to guy. In the back seat are some refreshments (two bottles of Fanta Orange, one bottle of water, some nuts, and a package of M&Ms to be exact) and a stack of newspapers with the Edwards' pictures plastered on the front under headlines announcing the return of the cancer and his decision to carry on with the presidential campaign.

A plane lands and taxis into its parking spot. I am waved over.

I am nervous. More nervous than I was when I allowed my pledge sister to kiss me. More nervous than the night I lost my virginity.

"Hi," I say, as Sen. and Mrs. Edwards enter the car and John Davis introduces me to them. "Nice to meet you."

Elizabeth immediately picks up the papers and starts to flip through the headlines. I think she's about to say something about the cancer, about how hard the last week has been for her, maybe even break down in tears, instead all she can muster is, "God, I look fat here."

I smile and then she apologizes to me, "I'm sorry. We're not normally this vain. Please ignore us. Thank you so much for driving."

"Don't worry about it," I say. "It's no problem."

She reminds me of my own mother, with her soft calming voice. And I want to say something nice, something heartfelt, but what do you say to the woman you barely know who has just found out she's dying? A woman whose husband also happens to be vying for the shot at becoming the Democratic presidential candidate.

If it were later, I would have been better at this. I would've known that anything nice, even a simple "I'm sorry to hear the news" would do. Because I would've been through the same thing. I would've known what it felt like to have people know you're facing a tough disease and have them say nothing. Or inappropriate things. Like when I first heard my own bad news, and Jay, the guy I was casually dating, called to tell me that Mercury was in retrograde and the planets were misaligned and he was quite certain that my neurologist was crazy and most likely all the pain and numbness that was wreaking havoc on my body was caused by the stars and I'd be better soon.

I would've known that silence was the worst. But I don't. I hadn't learned those lessons yet.

So I take the Edwards to their hotel on Pico, the only nice one in the area that is unionized and I tell them I'll be back in a while to drive them to the fundraising event that night.

But just half an hour later, I am summoned back to the hotel. Mrs. Edwards, and the woman who has been hired to oversee the campaign's fundraising in LA, need me to take them shopping.

I drive them to trendy Montana Avenue, where the hot moms of Santa Monica shop for designer baby clothes and gowns of their own.

I ask Mrs. Edwards what kind of clothes she is looking for and she replies, "Something up to date, but something that a first lady could wear." She puts on her shades and for a second I feel like I am sitting next to Jackie O. And it hits me, this is for real. This woman could actually be the first lady one day. And here I am driving her around in a rented car wearing something from Banana Republic.

But the worst part is, when she can't find anything that looks nice enough or that would be appropriate for the event that evening, I still can't find anything to say that seems right. All I can think about is here's a woman who has just found out she is dying, who is hoping her husband will be president one day, and I can't even find her a store where she can buy a nice outfit.

In the backseat of the car, Elizabeth gets on her cell phone and dials the campaign office. "Someone needs to help me pack next time. Or at least keep me better informed as to what events I will be attending. I can't be out shopping two hours before I'm supposed to be somewhere."

Her soft exterior starts to crack and I can sense her anger as she continues to reprimand some young college intern on the other end of the call.

I almost want to cry. Because inside, I know that in some way I have failed her. As a woman, I understand. In some inherent way, I get that this isn't about the clothes. This is about finding something that makes you feel good, in a time when everything feels wrong. After my diagnosis, I would really get it. And I would've responded appropriately. But now I can only remain silent. I am just a volunteer who is in denial that something is wrong with her own body.

In hindsight, I would have had plenty to say. I could've bonded with her. I would've known what was right. I wouldn't have been so timid. When John Edwards announced in January of 2008 that he was dropping out of the race, all I could think about was, *Is Elizabeth okay?* I could care less about the politics or the future of America. Everything became about the person.

I've watched my own priorities start to shift from career, money, and success to family, health, and happiness and I want to relive my political experience all over again.

I want to do it right.

Months later, when I think about that night, when the who's who of Hollywood gathered to hear John and Elizabeth give their speeches and the press and paparazzi hung around the perimeter of Heather Thomas's sprawling property, all I could do is play it back the way I wish it had been. I imagine myself being bolder, needing more answers from the man who wants to be President.

When Senator Edwards finishes his speech, and turns the microphone over to the audience to ask him about healthcare and poverty, the war in Iraq, and the future of the US, I imagine I would step right up and ask my own questions.

"Senator Edwards," I'd begin. "I don't know much about politics, but there is something I believe only you can answer." Then I'd launch into my speech. The things that concern my world. "Mr. Edwards, had you known that your wife would get cancer, would you have married her? If, when you were in your twenties, she told you she knew this would happen, would you have continued the relationship or even began it in the first place? Because, Mr. Presidential Hopeful, I wonder the same things right now. I wonder if I tell the guy I'm dating that I most likely have MS, is he going to run? I wonder who's going to want to love me. I wonder who's going to take me for sickness and health when they know the sickness is inevitable. That there's a huge probability that I will one day end up in a wheelchair wearing diapers. I wonder, Mr. Husband of a woman who is dying, if you would do it all over again. I wonder, even if you knew all the heartache, would you still fall in love? Because Mr. Democrat, I am a girl who needs to know. Who needs to know if a man will ever fall in love with her, despite her condition. Who will stand by her side through everything. I need to know, Mr. Father of Four Children, if you would still have this family, knowing that one day soon you will be the only parent in your children's lives. I need to know that someone will take me and fulfill my dream of motherhood, knowing that one day things could get hard, that I might not be as useful as I am now. That I might not be able to play kickball in the yard with my kids, that I might be unable to brush my daughter's hair, or tie my son's tie. I need to know, John Edwards, that there are men out there who can see beyond all this. That there are men who won't leave or stray when things get tough. Who can love no matter what. Who can love me. Forever. But most of all, I need to know. Can a Democrat really change my world?"

Chapter Nine

THE SECRET

M y very first boyfriend almost died on my lips.
I was 14 and in complete and utter love. It was a
Saturday night and we had been making out on my parents'
grey leather sofa in the living room when his eyes began to
roll back into his head and he became unresponsive.

I started to panic.

I'd read *Dear God, It's Me Margaret* and practiced kissing
for two years on my index and middle fingers, but no one
had warned me that this could happen.

I tried to wake him, but he wouldn't wake.

I shook him, but he wouldn't move.

I kissed him, but his mouth was dry.

This could not be the way it was supposed to go.

Had I stuck my tongue in too far? Maybe I was supposed
to touch "it." Had I exhausted him?

I called upstairs for help and my mom came running
down. She took one look at me then looked at Jason and
called for my dad.

My hands started to shake. If it were enough for my
mom to call in my dad, then clearly I had done something
wrong.

"Were you guys drinking? Did you take any drugs?"
she asked.

"No. No," I immediately responded. "I don't know what's wrong with him," I continued, then wondered if maybe he had taken some kind of drug. But I was just a freshman in high school. I didn't even know anyone who did drugs. Where would he have gotten them from?

"What were you guys doing?" my mom asked.

"Uh, uh…"

"You have to tell us," my dad said.

"We were just kissing. And then he stopped. And then he wouldn't talk," I said. "I don't know what's wrong with him," I repeated.

"Let me try," my dad said.

He stood next to Jason and shouted his name as he grabbed his shoulders and tried to wake him. But again nothing happened.

"I'm calling 911," my mom said as her hands turned shaky with fear.

As she dialed, I stood by Jason's side and my dad, who's normally soft spoken and laid back continued to attempt to shake Jason awake as he barked louder and louder, "Jason. Jason. Jason!"

My dad turned to me. "Are you sure he didn't take anything?"

All I could do was nod and whisper, "I'm sure."

Jason's skin was pale. His body was limp.

My mom finally hung up the phone. "The ambulance is on its way. Gary, go see if his dad is here to pick him up yet."

My dad got up and quickly went out the front door. When the door closed, the gates opened to my emotions and my eyes filled with tears.

"It's going to be okay," my mom said as she took my hand and held it up to Jason's face. "Can you feel that? He's breathing. He'll be all right. Maybe he ate something bad."

I nodded, okay. I had to believe my mom. Then I kept my hand close to his face and continued to watch his chest rise and fall in a slow shallow rhythm.

You can't die, I thought. *I'm only a kid. We're in love. We have plans for the future. Remember? I'm going to go to college in California. You're going to follow me. I'm going to lose my virginity to you. We're going to get married. We're going to have kids. A house. A life together.*

You. Can. Not. Die.

"We need juice, do you have any juice?" a voice shouted.

I quickly pulled my hand away from Jason's barely shaven face as his dad came rushing into the room.

"He's diabetic," he said as my mom hurried to the fridge and poured a giant glass of orange juice.

"You didn't know, did you?" he turned and asked me.

I shook my head no.

"He's embarrassed," Jason's dad said.

My mom then returned with the juice and Jason's dad attempted to pour some into Jason's mouth. "We had no idea. I should have given this to him earlier," my mom said.

"He'll be okay, once we get some sugar in him," Jason's dad calmly responded.

Jason's dad remained calm, but Jason's mouth wasn't moving and the juice was pouring down his chin. The sugar was never going to get into his bloodstream.

"Is there anything else we can give him? A shot of insulin or glucose, or something? My grandfather was diabetic," my mom said as an explanation.

"I don't have any of that on me. Jason. JASON!"

Now Jason's dad started to shake him and call out his name and I got the sense that things were getting more urgent, that without sugar or help or something, Jason might just slip away.

I stepped back from the couch and let his dad continue to try and wake him as my mom grabbed a hold of my hand and squeezed it tight.

"The paramedics are on the way," my dad reiterated in an effort to keep everyone calm, but I was no longer calm.

Thoughts of the movie *My Girl* ran through my head. What if my only love, my best friend, died? How could I go on living? How would I ever find love again? I would be the girl everyone talked about. The one who had lost her soul mate. The one who was all alone.

Waaaahhhhaaa, waaaahhaaa, the sirens finally blared down the street and my dad opened the door and ushered in the paramedics.

They immediately went to work.

Needles went into Jason's arm. Sensors went onto his chest. Blood splattered on the leather couch and the four of us stood back and watched.

My eyes stared intently and I studied the paramedics' every move. As a kid I loved *Rescue 911* and any other medical show I could find, the more real it was the better. But this was a tad too real for me. I started to turn away, but then I saw Jason's eyes begin to flutter.

Jason was alive.

The tragedy was averted. I would not end up alone.

"Where's Cory?" he asked.

I reached out and grabbed his hand.

After he finally came all the way to, the paramedics took Jason to the hospital for further observation and I kissed him good night.

Jason's dad thanked my parents for being so responsive and helpful and then he left with his son in the ambulance.

When our front door shut I broke into tears. My parents held me as I cried for all the things I thought I was going to lose.

That Monday at school Jason gave me a letter, which I recently found in an old box of things at my parents' house.

Here is what it said:

Who knows what could've happened if you gave up? Well, I know, but I don't think you want to know. They say after it happens the first time, it gets worse the next and becomes less noticeable when it starts.

Diabetic shock had changed our lives. From that day forward Jason and I had a teenage love that was like no other. In some way, I had saved his life and no matter how messed up our young relationship became, we would forever be bonded in a unique way. Together we had seen that love carries the possibility of loss and that image of his limp body on my parents' couch would never be erased from my mind.

For two years we continued to profess our love for each other and plan a future with our young hearts, but like most first loves, things didn't work out between the two of us. Our relationship ended our sophomore year of high school and during our junior year Jason and his family moved to Georgia and I never saw him again. We sent letters here and there, but by the time I went away to college in LA we had completely lost touch.

Over the years, I often wondered what happened to him. After all that I'd seen that one Saturday evening I think I always feared that he wouldn't be around very long, but I never let my mind go to that dark place. I only wondered, where did he go to college? Did he ever get married? Does he have kids? What does he do for a living? What's he like as an adult? Would we still get along? Would we laugh about our crazy teenage love and the heartaches we put each other through?

When Facebook came out, I tried to find him, but no profile under his name showed up and I never looked for him again. I figured he was living his life and I mine and if we ever met once more we'd have drinks and talk about the past, laughing about how everything was so dramatic with us and how we thought we couldn't live without each other. I'd read him all the letters I'd found at my parents' and we'd reminisce about how we used to sneak around the school to kiss in darkened hallways.

Whenever someone asked me about my first love, I always told the story of Jason.

The other night my friend Jen and I were talking about the fact that it's hard to meet decent guys in LA. We started telling stories of our past relationships and I told her about Jason.

Jen is a diabetes educator and works for a company that produces insulin pumps, so I asked her, "Do you think he's okay?"

"I'm sure. Do you know how good they are now at managing the 'betes?"

"Yeah, I guess you're right," I said.

We ordered another glass of wine and enjoyed the rest of our evening, but for some reason I couldn't get Jason out of my mind.

So when I got home I Googled something.

Jason _____ Georgia obituary.

And there it was.

The truth.

My first love was gone.

He'd passed away less than a year before. He had no wife and no kids and there was no explanation for his death except that donations could be made in his name to the Juvenile Diabetes Research Foundation.

I started crying. He was only 29. He'd never married. He'd never had the life we'd imagined.

Then I started thinking, what if we'd never broken up? What if he had come to California with me? What if we'd gotten married? What if we'd had kids?

I wouldn't be worried about the fact that I was still single.

I would be a widow.

But…

I would have found love. I would have gotten married. When I'd been told I had MS, he would've been there. I wouldn't have had to wonder whether anyone would ever love me despite my disease. He would have already taken me in sickness and in health. We would've had no secrets.

I know it's a cliché, but is it better to have loved and lost or to have never loved at all?

I don't know.

But I did find this at the end of Jason's letter:

*Loving you **only** for the rest of eternity, forever and ever, caring for you only, for the rest of my life (and then some).*

And I guess now I hope that the words he wrote were true, that at 14 Jason knew he would reach heaven before me and I would forever have someone else watching over me, caring for me for the rest of his life, *and then some,* because lord knows I could use the help.

Chapter Ten

GOLDEN SHOWERS

I now have a fear. Wizz. Urine. Pee. Number one. I don't care what you call it. Piss scares the crap out of me.

Here's why.

I have an appointment to see the MS specialist in December, but for these next four weeks I'm back to waiting, and playing medical detective.

I am sitting at my computer at home. The Writer's Guild has recently declared a strike on the Alliance of Motion Picture and Television Producers and there is not much work to be done. In a few months the strike will be over and I'll be back to researching things like cocaine overdoses, or reading scripts based on famous comic books, and giving notes on big blow-'em-up scenes. Today, however, I am on a mission to sort out all of the possible symptoms of MS.

Two days ago I had gone to the library and checked out Montel Williams's memoir on dealing with MS and found two other books from famous people living with the disease: Squiggy, from *Laverne and Shirley,* and Richard Cohen, talk show host Meredith Vieira's husband. I wanted to read people's firsthand experiences with the symptoms, to see if I could gain any insight.

This morning I had finished reading all 700-and-some-odd pages of those three books. I poured over every word, looking for some semblance to my life. Unfortunately, all of these guys' experiences were different. No one had my story. There was nothing I could compare myself to or relate to, and I found myself at a dead end.

So now I am on the MS Society's website, looking at this whole situation in a much more methodical way. I sit up straight at my desk, click on the button labeled *Symptoms* and start to make notes.

On a pad of paper, I make a list and separate it into columns.

There is a column of my past issues…

Fatigue, pain, depression

My current situation…

Numbness, memory loss, spasticity

The future that lies ahead…

Difficulty walking, vision problems

And my new fixation…

Incontinence, sexual dysfunction

Which is why I now fear the yellow. Incontinence and sexual dysfunction? What the hell?

This is a giant curveball in my understanding of the disease. The neurologist never spoke of pissing my pants and none of those old dudes talked about this shit in their books. This is like a whole new world that I'm not sure I'm ready to enter.

When I was 17, a group of us were out on a boat on a Saturday night. It was a small speedboat that one of my friend's family owned for water skiing. They lived in a neighborhood with a series of lakes and rivers. Over one of those lakes there was a bridge. It was common for high school students to jump off the middle of the bridge as a teenage rite of passage. That night, there were about six of us on the boat, one of whom had won the state championship in diving several years in a row. When we pulled up close to the bridge, my friends started jumping off the back of the boat. I was a strong swimmer, so I figured I would go last. The night was dark, the water was darker. "Get off already," the driver shouted. Despite the fact that we had drifted closer to shore, I figured all was good and without a second thought I tucked my shins underneath me and jumped into the water. It was a cool summer night, but the impact burned like the sun. My shins slammed against a pile of rocks as I heard my friends scrambling up the embankment to get to the bridge. I gasped in pain. I had jumped into a foot of water. "Come on, Cory," they screamed back at me. I closed my eyes and held in the terror. "Go ahead without me," I managed. As they made their way to the top of the bridge, I slowly made my way back to the boat. I lifted myself onto the back ledge and found a bloody and bruised mess upon my legs. I took a towel and wrapped myself in it as I sat shivering in my underwear. The driver apologized. I said it wasn't his fault. I'd be fine. My friends took spectacular dives from above. I could not watch as they sprung from the concrete ledge, because I feared what was underneath. Later we laughed about my mishap, and I kept the severity of my injuries hidden. I did not want to be the buzzkill to that teenage night, and I never wanted to jump into the unknown again.

But now here I am staring at a list of symptoms.

The pad of paper filled with my notes is a scribbled mess. It's a pile of rocks waiting to slam into my body and the only thing I can decipher in the black ink is the fact that my sleuthing is a list of possibilities, but no certainties. It's like MS is the snowflake of diseases, showering down a bunch of unique symptoms, until you can't handle them anymore, quickly turning into an avalanche that covers you in a solid pocket of ice, withholding air until you suffocate under its pressure.

I take a deep breath.

I want to forget what I've read, but the problem with this idea is that I have already pulled back the curtain of knowledge and I now know what may lie ahead; and it doesn't look good.

A future filled with love and success? Please. It's more like there will be a day when I'm peeing my pants, unable to reach orgasm.

When they say, "Hey, kid you've got a bright future ahead of you," I'll now have to turn and laugh, "Ha! Only if said future includes golden showers and a bright pink vibrator." Because that's what I'm looking at. That's how bright the future's going to be for this kid.

I stand up from my desk and start to wander my room out of frustration. How am I going to get through this last bit of discovery?

I grab my *Multiple Sclerosis for Dummies* book in a last ditch attempt to find hope, but the advice they give and the stories they tell are all the same when it comes to incontinence. *Talk with your partner, they'll understand. Bob and I have learned to laugh at my "accidents."* And: *Ted and I have known each other for 50 years, we've had three kids, seven grandkids, and lived through the depression; we've seen worse. This has even made our marriage stronger.*

Therein lies the real problem.

You see, none of this is one bit helpful for someone who is 28 and single. Because, I guarantee you, unless I can find some kinky freak, there is no guy who's going to find my pissing all over him attractive. No matter how *accidental* it is.

A golden shower, as I've heard this "accident" called, is not on the top of most guys' list of things to do before they die. Sex in an elevator. Sex on a plane. Road head. Threesome. These? All men's fantasies. And what girl doesn't feel like their only purpose on this planet is to fulfill every man's sexual desire?

Which is why I now find myself in an even bigger conundrum. Because, if I follow the three-date rule, and sleep with whomever I'm dating on our third date, I run the risk of blowing my cover. Let's say I take said date home with me, or he takes me back to his place. We start kissing, necking, even heavy petting, but if we move on to the intercourse, the unpredictability of this disease could kick in and I may just have an "accident." Thereby outing myself and inadvertently disclosing the fact that I am sick. I suppose I could lie and say that I'm really into fetish sex. Maybe even offer up my breasts as targets for him to take aim and fire a stream of urine. But I don't believe you should build a relationship on dishonesty.

So now I need a new rule of three: Keep your legs shut and do not reveal the MS until you've been dating for at least three months. No sex until the guy knows the real you.

I make a mental note of this as I flop down on my bed and contemplate the realities of this rule.

Three months is usually a safe zone. The zone where you've already gotten through the basic get-to-know-yous, and you've moved on to more serious topics. Topics like how crazy your family is, or your plans for the future: Do you see yourself married? Do you want kids? The way I see it, if you're willing to reveal this much, it's probably an appropriate time to reveal the MS.

Usually, you're pretty invested in the relationship by this point and most guys don't take off running. But now as I lie here alone on top of my fluffy comforter, a list of symptoms drawn out on the desk in the corner, I realize that like all rules in life, there are exceptions.

My exception? Brad. Brad and I had been dating for around eight months when I was first referred to the neurologist. I thought about not telling Brad anything, after all we hadn't known each other that long. However, when I was super quiet at dinner one night and he asked what was wrong, I told him that I had to see a neurologist the following week.

"Oh my gosh," he said. "Well, if you need anything, I'm here for you."

"I'm sure it's nothing," I said. "But thanks for the offer."

I'm obviously not the type who likes help, so while his offer was sweet, I wasn't about to take him up on it. I could do this on my own.

We went back to eating and I truly thought it was nothing. That I would go to the neurologist, she'd tell me I was fine, and I'd be on my way. Of course, that was not the case.

So, when I had to get the MRI of my brain and my neurologist offered me some Valium to take before the test to ease the anxiety, I happily accepted, until she told me that I would need someone to drive me to and from my appointment and then the real anxiety hit.

I had to ask for help.

I gathered up my courage and asked Brad if he would do it. I was relieved when he said he would, and thought how great it was that I'd finally found a nice guy to date.

But the day before my appointment…

"So, can you pick me up at ten?" I asked.

"Um…"

"Did you forget?"

"Actually, I told my dad I'd play in this golf thing with him."

"Oh." I stopped right there. *Hold in the tears.* But I couldn't do it. I was already worn down. I had been living with the news that there was most likely something wrong with me and this MRI was supposed to help determine exactly what. I heaved my tears at Brad. Each drop a punch to his gut. Then I looked up at him through glassy eyes and had one thought, *You are not the one.*

Mental note: If you want to know if someone's right for you, ask them to be there for you in a real time of crisis.

On the other hand, if you want to start to doubt your past relationship decisions, call your super nice ex-boyfriend, the one you once lived with, and ask him to drive you to and from your MRI because you're going to be too high to do it yourself, and he will be right there by your side.

Some girls return to their exes for "free" sex, I return to mine in a crisis. It's too bad he and I don't still have the same chemistry we once did. Otherwise, I wouldn't need any of these crazy rules.

And I definitely wouldn't have to think about the fact that one day I may have to tell the man I'm with that because of the MS I just may pee on him. I'm hoping this day never comes, or at least comes when I'm like 80 and I've been married for 50 years and my husband's already in diapers himself and we're barely even able to have sex once a year. But if it comes before then, I guess now I'm prepared.

Chapter Eleven

TWELVE STEPS

Screw doctors. Everything I need to know about how to handle this disease, I learned from an alcoholic.

First: Wine, beer, and shots rock. You can blame everything on them.

Second: The more damaged you are, the more people want to help.

And third: I'm dying.

But before I get into all that you should know about my special alcoholic. Let's call him Chuck. I call him that because that's how he makes me feel, and why call him anything else?

Chuck and I met through mutual friends. At the time, he was living in San Francisco, and though I found him attractive and a fun guy to hang out with, I didn't think much of it because he lived so far away. But a year later, when Chuck moved to Newport Beach for work, we started dating.

Our first month together was a whirlwind. Things were great. We were in the honeymoon phase of new coupledom and nothing could take us down. We were falling in love quickly and I had even had the thought that he could be the one.

I was just waiting for him to say the three magic words…

And there is never a more appropriate time to tell some-one you love them than when you are completely shit-faced.

I was sitting in the galley of my friend's boat on the built in couch, as the engine of the 42-foot cruiser roared over the waves from Catalina Island back to Newport Harbor. Chuck was wasted, dozing in and out of consciousness as he buried his head between my breasts. The shots of tequila made him look like a mouse fresh out of the womb, looking for anything that might provide him sustenance. I brushed his sweaty hair from his forehead and looked at him with a smile. *Shit,* I thought, *we've all been there.* I can recount plenty of college stories that would make this moment look normal. There was the time I danced on a table at Miyagi's, the time I skinny-dipped in Hermosa, the time I...

Suddenly, Chuck burst into consciousness, looked at my bosom and said it. "I love you."

"I love you too," I responded without a second thought. I wanted to kiss him. Have him look into my eyes, and say it again. But his eyes quickly floated and bobbled back into his head, completely unaware of his surroundings.

I let out a small laugh and brushed it off. Chalked the experience up to another drunken moment. I guess when you're 31, like Chuck, these things still happen.

Soon, night began to fall and we were back on dry land. At Chuck's apartment, I thought things were going to turn sober.

We decided to order some dinner. Because he was able to tell me what he wanted, I assumed he was no longer inebriated and was ready to talk when I hung up the phone with the pizza guy.

"Hey, so you know I had to take care of you on the boat today?"

"What?" he asked.

"Yeah, you fell down the stairs and Darrin sent me in to look after you."

"No I didn't," he argued. But then he looked down at his knee and saw a giant bruise covered in scrapes and decided to stay quiet.

"You were a little bit out of control. It was kind of embarrassing since Emily's mom was there."

"Embarrassing?"

"A little bit."

"Now I'm embarrassing to be with?" he shouted, some sort of switch beginning to flip in his head. And I quickly realized I was wrong. He was not sober. The man was still drunk.

"I didn't say you were embarrassing. I was talking about the situation," I said cautiously.

"Oh, is that so? How about this?" he opened up a drawer in the kitchen and slammed it shut. The sound a mighty slap against the air-conditioned air.

"What are you doing?"

"Just showing you," he said angrily as he opened up a cabinet and proceeded to slam it shut. I could see the anger boil up inside him, the alcohol still running through his veins.

"Seriously, what are you doing?" I asked. But he didn't respond. Just continued to move through the kitchen, opening and slamming shut every door and drawer.

"Stop!"

He paused and looked at me with glassy eyes.

He took a two-by-four that was sitting in the hallway and held it up for me to see. I turned my head as he threw the board against the wall. The drywall crumpled underneath the force. My body slid down my chair.

He pounded the wall with his fists.

I clenched my own, waiting for the moment to end. The room got silent. And then…

"Come here," Chuck said. I looked up at him, my eyes filled with tears. He saw this and his anger quickly ceased. "I'm sorry. Don't cry. You know I'd never hurt you."

I hesitated. I didn't want to move and I didn't want to say anymore, lest I set off another tirade, and release Jekyll or Hyde—whichever one is the evil one.

"Tell me that you know I won't hurt you."

I nodded slowly.

"Good. Because I love you." He grabbed me into his arms.

"I love you too," I said. I wanted to tell him that he just scared the hell out of me, but all I could think was that I was happy that the alcohol hadn't blacked out the memory of those three words and he still loved me.

I snuggled into his chest and made a promise to myself, if it happened again I'd leave him. But this was easier said than done and Chuck and I continued our relationship for seven more months before it all came to a head at my 27th birthday and he ended up drunkenly making out with another woman. I finally told him he had a drinking problem and I could no longer be with him.

Luckily, it was over, but I had learned some things from this alcoholic. All the mental abuse I put up with? Completely worth it.

Here's the ironic thing. Chuck's mom has MS and according to Chuck she is dying. In fact, this was what he used to pull at my heart and get me to forgive him.

"My mom is dying," he'd say. "That is why I drink so much. That is why I want to escape."

At the time, I knew nothing about MS. All I knew was that it made you wheelchair-bound. Whatever Chuck told me I believed. If he said his mom was dying, then she was. Of course, I now know that MS is debilitating, but it doesn't kill. In fairness, I do know that his mom's MS has progressed and that she is of the generation that was not offered any of the disease modifying drugs, simply because they were not around. I know that she is far worse off than I am today and I pray that she is still doing well and that even though she is in a wheelchair, she will continue to live a happy and fulfilling life, with no further medical complications.

But when I found out that I, too, had to face the disease, all I could think was I'm dying, and Chuck has it easy. After I broke things off with him, he decided to work on getting rid of his disease. Twelve months later, he was getting his one-year chip from AA and I was being pelted with bad news.

While he gets to brag to our mutual friends how he's beating his disease, all I get to tell my friends is that I've been told I have a new disease.

There's a part of me that wants to go on a week-long bender, get completely sauced, do totally inappropriate things, and have someone come to my rescue. Tell me that I have a problem, and force me to start attending AA meetings.

If dealing with a disease were that easy, I would give anything to have the alcoholism instead of this damn MS. I want to go to a meeting and get cured. I don't want to have to keep praying that I can walk. I want to be able to take things day by day. Wake up each morning and have my only worry with the disease be that I shouldn't drink today, not whether

I can still feel my toes. I want someone to give me a little chip for every 30 days I make it without any progression of the disease. I don't want to have to keep getting MRIs to see how much damage my brain has accumulated. I want to stand up in front of a crowd and say, "Hi, I'm Cory and I'm an alcoholic." Not have to wonder who I should tell, or if I should tell at all, or when I should tell someone that I'm facing a life with MS.

But, I'm not an alcoholic so that fantasy will have to end right there.

However, that doesn't mean that I can't pretend to have some sort of addiction and take to ordering an Effen vodka on the rocks every time I go out. So when I start speaking and my words get jumbled or I stop mid-sentence because I have no clue what the hell I'm talking about, I can just take a sip of my drink and let others wonder… can you really get drunk off of two sips of vodka?

I'll smile and flip my hair, letting them think I really like to drink, but I won't tell the truth. I won't tell anyone that I have a disease that has now affected my cognition and I'm not as smart as I used to be.

Instead, I'll just blame it on the booze.

Chapter Twelve

THE RULES

R ule number one: Do not wear a thong to the doctor's office.

Just don't. No matter how loud your mother's voice is screaming at you to wear your clean, pretty underwear in case you get hit by a car, or washed down a river. Don't do it. Wear your granny panties. Wear your little lace hot pants that cover your ass. But don't wear your thong.

I found this out the hard way.

In December 2007, I finally got in to see the MS specialist. My parents flew out from Chicago and accompanied me to the appointment with the hope that the specialist would say the neurologist was out of her mind. Unfortunately, she didn't give me any better news. She, too, believed it was MS and, in an effort to determine whether or not her gut reaction to my case was correct, ordered another series of tests. According to her, she needed one more piece of clinical evidence to officially give me the MS diagnosis. My parents returned home somber just before the holidays, and I went in for the test.

This test was called an *evoked potential*. When I called to schedule the appointment, they told me to wear comfortable clothes. So I put on my favorite yoga pants, a T-shirt, covered my newly highlighted hair with a newsboy cap and topped it all off with a jean jacket.

I thought I looked put together, but not trying too hard. After all, I was going to be spending the day getting poked and prodded and zapped with electric currents. But being the optimistic girl that I am, I had to look somewhat good. Hello? I was spending the day at the UCLA Medical Center. Alone. Do you know how many opportunities that allots me to get trapped in an elevator with Dr. McDreamy? Sixty-two. I calculated.

So, here I am waiting on the second floor of Building 300. The room is pretty empty except for an elderly married couple. I smile at them and they smile back. For a second I wish I had asked someone to come with me. But there is no time to feel sorry for myself because suddenly it is my turn.

"Ms. Martin," I hear my name called from around the corner. I walk toward the voice and nearly run straight into the technician. "Cory?" he asks.

I lift my head to reply but suddenly I am speechless.

Here's the thing about being 28 and going through all this medical hoopla. Doctors are no longer these older mythical figures. They are your peers.

And this technician? Hot. My age. And definitely someone I would talk to at a bar.

He gives me that look. That look that says: *You are not like the elderly people I usually see in here.* The look that says: *This could be fun.*

Ha!

Rule number two: Fun is not a medical term.

No matter how hot the guy poking and prodding you is, your appointment will never be fun.

I enter the tiny room. The technician, we'll call him Derek, sits me down in a chair in the corner.

He starts to explain the first test.

"I'm going to stick these sensors on your head and then you'll have to stare at this screen the entire time. Some people find it boring. A bit mesmerizing. But try not to fall asleep."

"No problem," I say. "So, how's your day?" I ask, trying to start up a conversation, anything to make this feel more normal.

"Good. And you?" he asks.

I try to think of a witty response, but I don't even get the chance because...

"Are you taping those to my head?" I ask as I hear him rip a piece of tape off the roll and quickly stick a sensor to my scalp.

"Uh, yeah, but I promise not to pull any of your hair out."

"I guess it's a good thing I don't have a hot date right after this," I joke.

He laughs. Then continues to tape sensors to the remaining areas of my head.

"All right. So, we're ready. You ready?"

"This isn't going to hurt is it?"

"No," he says. "You'll be fine." He squeezes my shoulder and lets his hand linger a bit longer than he probably should.

The test begins and, as told, I keep my eyes focused on the screen in front of me, but my mind starts to wander. I wonder how many other girls my age have been through here? Did he place his hand on their shoulders? I wonder if he's ever hit on any of them? I wonder if I could hit on him? Is that against hospital policy? Emily Post never mentioned any rule about hitting on your technician, did she? I wish I had covered that zit on my chin...

"You still okay?" he asks, pausing between cycles of the test.

"Yeah," I smile. "I'm still good."

I look over at Derek. He smiles. I sit up straight, instinctively forcing my breasts to attention. Then I contemplate writing my number on my medical records. Or...

Maybe, when this is over, Derek will walk me to the elevator. He'll ask if he can push the button to the basement floor. I'll tell him he can push my button any time. He'll enter the cabin. The doors will shut. We'll descend down. I'll pull the emergency stop button. The alarm will sound. We'll make out until the police come. Then, when they go to arrest Derek, I can just explain how depressed I've been lately, dealing with the MS. I'll make a sad face and say that Derek was the only thing that's made me feel better in months. The cops will back away and Derek and I will walk off into the sunset.

I smile again at Derek. He smiles back. The connection is palpable. He gets up from his seat. *Oooh, he feels it too. I wonder if we could make out right here. The door is probably locked. If not, who cares?* He approaches. *Oh my God, is he going to make a move?*

"So, I need you to undress and put this on."

Huh? I stare back at him completely dumbfounded. I can't get naked now. I took a class on writing rom coms. This is not how it's supposed to go down.

"You can leave your underwear on. But I need to put the sensors on your spine, so you'll have to remove your bra."

My bra? What about the triumphant boy who likes to show off that he can unhook a girl's bra with one hand?

"I'll be back in a few minutes," he says then exits the room.

I start to take off my yoga pants and realize, oh my God, I am wearing my cotton blue striped thong that is way too big. I put on the gauzy hospital robe, open to the back as instructed. I tie the ties as tight as possible. Maybe Derek won't have to see the thong. I think I have to lie on that table over there anyway. The back won't even be open. He'll never see a thing. I finally convince myself this won't be that bad.

Derek knocks and I tell him I'm decent. Or as decent as one can be in a hospital gown.

"Wow, this is some outfit," I joke. "So, you need me to get on the table?"

"Actually," he says, "I have to place these on you first."

Derek then holds up what looks like a centipede—a thick wire with a hundred sensors for legs. "It's going to take me a while. If you could stand with your back to me, I can start putting them on."

I turn away, allowing Derek to have a full view of my backside. Thank God I tied that gown tight. I sigh a sigh of relief, but gasp when I feel Derek untie the ties. My entire gown falls open for all the world to see.

My blue thong hangs in the breeze of the air-conditioned room, and my white ass glistens under the fluorescent lights.

Why did I eat that Del Taco last night? The cheese has probably already curdled up beneath the skin of my left butt cheek and Derek is now staring at it in this bright light.

For a moment, Derek and I stop talking. Actually, I stop. Any flirting, real or imagined, ceases to exist. Now I am just another patient with another white butt, who's swollen and bloated from too much Del Taco and her period. And, oh my God, I hope my tampon string is not hanging out of my too-big thong.

I stand there for what seems like forever. Derek touches each one of my vertebrae before taping another sensor on it. Great. So, not only does Derek get to view me practically naked, but now he's got his hands all over me. This is so not how it happens on the big screen.

When Derek finishes, I am finally allowed to lie on the table.

"Now, I'm going to put these electrical shocks on your hands and when your fingers start moving on their own, I'll know I've got it at the right voltage."

"Voltage?" I ask. This does not sound good.

"More like an electrical current. It shouldn't be that strong."

"Is this going to be like that ab machine thing that shocks your muscles into shape?" God bless the infomercial for keeping a girl informed.

He laughs. "Sort of. Maybe a bit more."

"Okay, fine, do it," I say. I'm lying prone on the bed. My hands hooked to electrical charges and my spine covered in sensors that were so carefully placed by Derek himself while he got to take in my nakedness. "No, stop," I yell before he's even turned the thing on. I feel like a virgin waiting to get poked for the first time. What if it hurts? What if I scream out I love you on accident?

"Just tell me when."

"Okay, go. No. Wait. Okay. Go. No." We both start laughing. The connection comes back. "Okay. Go. No wait." He really starts laughing.

"I promise. It won't hurt."

He turns on the machine. The electric current surges through me. My fingers start to move on their own.

Ouch. Oh, crap. I LOVE YOU!

Rule number three: Never shout I love you prematurely.

Okay, so I didn't really say I love you. But I might as well have. The guy's seen more of me than any man has in a while.

The moment is awkward.

So I do the only thing I know how to do in this situation. I get to know him.

"So, how did you get into this field?" I ask, hoping he'll say something that validates the lovey-dovey thoughts in my head.

"Med school was too long and too hard, but I always loved medicine, so I figured this was the next best thing."

Lovely. McDreamy couldn't even cut it at med school. Maybe next he'll tell me he still lives at home.

Chapter Thirteen

KNOCKED UP

"I just want to get knocked up," I tell my mom over the phone as I flip through the marijuana cookbook she put in my stocking this year. Sugar cookies, mac 'n' cheese, honey pumpkin bread, who knew cannabis was like the butter of drugs?

"Or maybe you can just be one of those women who carries people's babies when they are incapable," she replies, taking the humanitarian approach to my newest thought on how to cure this chronic disease of mine.

"Kind of like killing two birds with one stone. Putting my MS into remission and bringing some joy to a young childless family. I like it," I reply, laughing on the inside because I think she thinks I'm joking. And there certainly is a part of me that thinks this would be a funny way to tell Randy, the guy I've been seeing since Brooke's wedding, that I have MS… *So I have this disease and the only cure is pregnancy, what do you say we go upstairs and do it?* But in reality there's some truth behind my madness.

In everything that I've read about MS, pregnancy just happens to be one of the best things for it. Apparently, the woman's body produces some hormone that forces the disease into remission, not permanently, of course, but for the nine months. So now, all the top doctors and scientists are trying to figure out how to replicate that hormone so that those of us who suffer from the disease can be free and clear from its debilitating effects.

In the meantime, however, I'm taking science into my own hands. Turning every single girl's worst nightmare into my dream. Luckily, the genes are stacked in my favor because fertility runs in the family. My grandma had 12 kids, her sister had eight, a couple aunts were married shotgun style, and there're a few distant relatives who doctored their marriage certificates so that their children would never know the truth behind their existence.

Oh, and then there are my parents.

Gary and Petey (real name Therese, but her dad wanted a boy so she got Petey as a nickname). They met when they were 15, sophomores at Lincolnway High School in New Lenox, Illinois. Mom was a cheerleader and Dad was a hockey-player-slash-golfer who smoked a lot of pot. Actually, I don't know that last bit for a fact, but I'm guessing by the long hair in the pictures and the story of the cheerleading coach who warned my mom to stay away from that Martin boy that there was definitely some pot being smoked. And maybe some acid under the tongue, but I don't know.

However, I have seen *Dazed and Confused* and *That '70s Show*, and I do know what people did back then. Plus, there's the roach clip my sister found in my mom's jewelry box when we were in high school. The thing was handcrafted of metal. There was a naked man and woman sculpted on the ends so that when you slid them into the 69 position the metal ends grabbed onto the joint. It's freaking genius, I must say. My mom obviously thought so too, because that's why, after all these years, she still has the "piece of art" her friend made her in shop class.

But enough about the pot. This is about more serious business. This is about me. How I came to exist in this world and how I know that I must certainly be just as fertile as all the other women who have popped out kids before me.

Mom and Dad dated all through high school. Even went to the senior prom together. The picture of them at the "Nights in White Satin" dance is so aptly placed on my bookshelf—right in front of Erica Jong's *Fear of Flying,* and right next to the picture of me, at three, reading *Playboy* with my dad.

I wonder now if my mom would've changed the three dating rules she had for me in high school: *No drinking. No drugs. No sex.*

Given the new circumstance of my health, I wonder if she'd tell my dates to give me a couple glasses of wine to get me loosened up then tell them to go make love to me like Jack to Rose on the Titanic.

Of course, I don't think my mom would really say these things, but the older she gets the more and more she becomes like her mom, Grandma Reed. And Grandma Reed was known for saying anything that popped into her head.

Like, I believe that when my dad showed up for the first time to take my mom to see Led Zeppelin, my grandmother told him, "Do not get Petey drunk, she gets romantic."

So what do you think my dad did next? Went out and bought a six-pack of course. Then held my mom's hand as Robert Plant sang *Heartbreaker.* Okay, so maybe he did more than hold her hand, but I'm not about to ask him. Quite honestly, I don't need to know, nor do I want that visual. It's nice enough to know that they still hold hands like they did back then. And I do believe they make out on occasion.

What's important is that there must have been something special between the two of them, because by the time they were juniors in college, things had gotten serious.

Mom was up in Vermont at St. Michael's College and Dad was at Temple University in Philadelphia. The year was 1978. It was Thanksgiving.

Dad caught a ride with some buddy who lived in the Northeast and got dropped off at Mom's brick and mortar dorm. I imagine that there was snow on the ground and there wasn't much to do except stay inside and do some more "hand-holding." Apparently, there must've been a lot of that going on because nine months later little old me was born. August 13, 1979. Six days before my dad turned 21 and five months after they got married.

Yes, in following tradition, Mom got knocked up, and she and Dad had a shotgun wedding.

The good news is, I always know what anniversary they're on by my age. Like this year, as I approach the big 2-9, they approach their 29th.

Now, here's something I must say about my existence. I did and do feel lucky to have been born to my parents. They gave me a lot of love and never made me feel like I was a mistake.

So, when I say that I want to get knocked up, I say it out of a place of love. I say it in the hopes that I can have the fairy tale that is my parents' marriage and the family that came out of it. Mom, Dad, me, and my little sister Cassie.

"Mom, when did Grandma have Uncle Tom?" I ask, inquiring about her youngest brother, my Grandma's 12th child.

"When she was 46," my mom replies.

"Great," I say with a smile, because, while I know that having a child would be great for my MS, it's not a guaranteed way to get rid of the Ms. in front of my name. So, it's good to know there's still time to find the one, get married, and then get knocked up. After all, fertility runs in the family. Now let's just hope *leprosy* doesn't, 'cause if it did, I really don't know who'd want to screw me then.

Chapter Fourteen

LIKE A VIRGIN

Lately, I've been thinking about becoming one of those born-again virgins. You know, the kind who feels like she's lost her innocence and decides to make a pledge to no longer have sex. Claiming that she's now waiting for marriage. Even taking it so far as to head on down to Beverly Hills so some plastic surgeon can rejuvenate her vagina, re-install her hymen, and plump her lips.

It's not that I've recently found God, or become some sort of super-slut that I feel bad. Nor do I actually need any of those aforementioned procedures.

It's just that I've reached a point where I've given up on sex.

It's not on purpose.

It's a boy. Randy.

We've gone out plenty. Made out bunches. Held hands in the theater and conversed over dinner. On our seventh date he brought me roses. There was and is promise with him. However, there is one problem with our dating and the reason why I'm having thoughts of becoming a born-again virgin. We've been seeing each other for some time now, and we have yet to sleep with each other.

Which, I know, is not the end of the world. And I have definitely been cautioned by my dad that "men aren't going to want to buy the cow, if they can get the milk for free."

And I do completely see his point. It's simple logic. The longer you hold out, the more the guy wants it. So, I have been holding out. However, there comes a time when it goes past the *I'm going to act innocent so this guy wants me,* phase and into the *Why the hell doesn't he want to sleep with me yet?* phase.

Which is the point I have now reached.

WHY WON'T THIS MAN RIP OFF MY CLOTHES?!

I'm wondering this as I lie topless in my bed with my jeans still on and Randy fully clothed. We're definitely making out, and if this were any other horny red-blooded American I've ever been with, he'd be ripping off his own clothes then tearing at my jeans and pulling at my panties. I would, of course, tell him to slow down, and then eventually after a few dates we'd get to the sex. But, this is Randy. And everything is different.

At first, I loved the fact that Randy wasn't like every other guy, pawing and clawing at me. I loved that I didn't have to keep saying "no" when I was trying to take things slow. And I loved the respect he showed for me. But come on now, it's been… one… two… three… It's been three months.

And aren't good things supposed to come in threes?

And isn't three… Oh. My. God.

Perhaps it's not Randy.

Perhaps it's me.

Coming back to bite myself in my own ass. My own three-month rule.

Randy still does not know about the MS and now we've hit the mark. That place where we've shared enough intimate facts about our lives that I should be able to tell him about this crazy ass disease that has me waking up in the middle of the night in pain. But I still haven't been able to tell him.

In fact, I don't even want to tell him. To be honest, I'm still in the denial phase of tragedy. Some days I don't even believe it's a fact of my life.

Maybe I'm hoping that if I never tell Randy the truth, this disease will never affect me. But now I'm starting to wonder… is *not* telling him starting to affect us?

What if I'm giving off the vibe of "please don't touch me," or "I'm waiting for marriage"?

I've certainly given off those vibes before. I used to be one of those good Catholic girls who thought she could save her virginity until marriage.

In high school, my friends used to tell all the boys that "Cory will suck, but she won't fuck."

Then all the kids in my class would have a good laugh at the expense of my virginity. But I held onto that thing for a while. I even thought I could make it through college without giving it up. Of course, that was not the case. I was miles away from home and anyone who knew me when I was the shy high school girl, and I was moving into my sexual prime. Once I turned 20, it was time to say good-bye to that virgin pledge I'd made to myself at 13.

Now that I'm older, I've had to create a whole new set of rules in an attempt to bring some sort of order to the chaos that is my health. And I wonder if, like in high school, these rules are putting a damper on my social life.

I wonder if I'm the one putting a halt on intimacy in my relationship with Randy.

I do believe the guy should make the first move when it comes to the sex, but I wonder if it's more than just me waiting for him to get the balls to strip me naked.

I wonder if he feels like there's something I'm not telling him. That maybe I have a giant secret that I have yet to whisper in his ear. That maybe it's plain and simple.

Randy is a genuinely good guy.

Not the type of guy who sticks his cock in any girl with a decent face and a perky pair of 34D breasts. Maybe, just maybe, Randy wants to get to know the real me, before we decide to get fully intimate. Maybe, this is our problem.

But now what?

Do I have to tell him the truth? Because I'm not so sure I'm ready for that. The last time I opened up about the possibility of my disease I found myself single yet again as Brad left me stranded with no ride to my MRI and Jay told me I was crazy, that my problems were based solely on the stars' misalignment.

How will I ever tell Randy?

It's not like I'm going to call him up and say, "You see, I have this three-month rule with men and it's time I told you I probably have MS, and I'm really hoping it doesn't freak you out, but if it does, you won't be the first guy to take off running, and I'm guessing you won't be the last."

No. That's not what I'm going to do. Instead I think I have to wait for the right moment. A point in time on one of our dates where I feel comfortable opening up to him.

Luckily, there's an upside to hopping into bed with a guy who's got rules on nakedness. When you spend most of your time making out like you're in seventh grade, you feel a hell of a lot less vulnerable when you're still wearing most of your clothes.

So, here we are again. In my bed, pretty much clothed, making out on top of my pink paisley sheets, when we take a break to lie there quietly in each other's arms and talk about the events of the past week.

Randy tells me how he had a physical that past Wednesday.

"I almost passed out," he says. "I hate needles and they had to draw blood."

"Was everything okay?"

"I'm as healthy as can be," he replies.

"Oh," I say softly, my mind spinning. *Here's my chance.* The topic of doctors is already on the table. I can simply lay it all out there.

"Um, speaking of doctors, there's something I need to tell you," I say, my voice shaking.

Randy pauses, then pulls away from me.

I realize now that while in bed it's probably not a good time to tell the guy you're with that there's something you need to tell him and it involves modern medicine. I'm sure he thought I was going to tell him I had chlamydia or crabs, HIV or syphilis.

"The doctors think I have MS," I finally blurt out.

"Oh," Randy says as his body unclenches from the fear of STDs I just inflicted upon him. "Okay."

"I wanted you to know, because I feel like I've been keeping a huge secret from you," I say softly as I clutch my down comforter.

"Thanks for telling me."

"You're welcome," I sigh.

"So, they caught it early? Right?"

"Yeah," I respond, knowing that that doesn't really make a huge difference in my prognosis unless I get on one of the drugs that is supposed to slow down the progression of the disease, but even that's not saying much. However, I do know that agreeing with him might make it easier for him to accept the truth of my situation.

"My pledge brother from college has it. He's not doing so well."

"I'm sorry to hear that," I say, also knowing full well that tomorrow morning I could wake up and fall into that "not doing so well" category.

"Well, I'm doing great," I say, pretending everything is perfectly fine with me and that I am far better off than his pledge brother.

"Good. I'm glad you shared that with me," Randy says as he squeezes me in for a hug and we fall back into the pillows on my bed and begin to kiss.

And I wish I could say that in celebration of my telling Randy about the MS, we stripped right down and did the dirty deed.

But we didn't.

And we still haven't. And now it's been five months since we began dating. And my friends joke that if Randy and I were to get married it would be totally appropriate for me to wear all white. And for a moment it's funny. But then it's not. Because now I'm concerned that maybe there's something bigger than my MS that is keeping us from having sex. Maybe it's a serious problem.

I decide to bring in the big guns.

My therapist.

Now, I know I haven't mentioned her before, and I had once been averse to therapy, but as you might imagine, a girl who's just been told she has an incurable disease would probably throw out her misconceptions and seek out the help of a mental health professional.

So, a month after the neurologist gave me the news, I decided to plop down on a comfy sofa and get myself analyzed.

The woman was great. She gave me a lot of insight into dealing with disease and the grief and depression that comes along with it. Talking to her definitely made all of the doctors' appointments and the stress of my changing life much easier, and I trusted her opinion. Once I was starting to feel sane again, I decided it was time to bring up the no sex with Randy thing, but what came out of her mouth was not what I expected.

When I finally told her about not having sex for five months and she asked the obligatory *Is he gay? Is he a virgin? Was he sexually abused?* questions and all the answers were no, she spent an entire hour trying to convince me that all I needed to do was take charge, grab Randy, "sit on him," then "ride him hard."

O-M-G!

First off, I don't want a woman who is older than my mother telling me I should ride anyone, especially not hard. Second, I didn't think therapists were supposed to convince you to do anything. And third, I don't want to ride him!

I don't want to ride him?

It's true. I don't want to ride him. Even though I thought that's what I wanted all along, it's not there. There's something missing. I can't make love to this man, because that's the girl I used to be. The girl who would want to sleep with a guy after they'd been dating three months. The girl who loved intimacy. The girl who longed for a loving touch. The girl who was healthy. The girl who...

No longer wants to have sex.

That is my new reality.

And I can tell you why. It's easy, really. With the MS in my life I no longer know who I am.

Because while my self-esteem is still very high and I don't look in the mirror and want to stop eating or start puking, my body image is destroyed. I have lost that utmost respect I used to have for my legs and my arms and my heart and my inner workings. The kind of respect the majority of us have, no matter if we're having a bad hair day or feeling bloated, because we can see what a miracle our daily functions really are.

After that therapy session, which was my last, I got the feeling this woman had never dealt with someone who was dealing with a disease that mangled or disabled their bodies. Because not once did she ever bother to ask me how I now felt about myself. My therapist never asked if I felt broken or damaged or betrayed by my body. All things you would expect someone to ask a girl who's facing a very uncertain future with the body her soul calls home.

I've read many articles lately about women who are battling breast cancer and after they've had their breasts removed feel incredibly damaged. I used to read the articles and sympathize, but I could never fully empathize. In my mind, I couldn't understand why a life saving surgery could traumatize one that much. But now? Now it is clear. It's about not feeling whole. About losing your sense of self. And, while I've never had to go through a surgery of that much change, I feel like I understand. Like in some ways, I am going through the same thing.

I may still have my breasts, but I no longer feel like a complete woman.

Because just like a woman who's had the outward symbol of her femininity taken away no longer feels like an object of sexual desire, I, too, no longer feel sexy.

I worry that if I ever do end up in a wheelchair, I will feel even shorter than I do now at five four. And there will be no way I can put on a pair of stilettos and stand tall, because I won't even be able to get up. I worry that when I'm curled up next to the man I'm with, he'll get frustrated with the fact that I have to keep moving around because I've got the worst feeling of pins and needles in my arms and legs and I have to pull away. And when the semi-numb patch on my back makes its way to my nether regions, and the question "is it in yet?" isn't a comment on the man's penis size, but a matter-of-fact question. I worry, how am I ever going to feel sexy again?

But above all else, I worry…

How am I ever going to stop feeling like a virgin? Not wanting to be touched for the very first time.

Chapter Fifteen

FAT TUESDAY

Before I ever got into swimming or practiced yoga, I was just a fat kid looking for her next sugar fix. I was one of those chunky little girls who got breasts before all the rest, because she had a few extra pounds above her mid-section. I loved ice cream and doughnuts and anything fried. I ate Cheez-Whiz on crackers and snuck cookies out of the kitchen cabinet. At nine years old, I weighed 100 pounds.

But there was no shame in my little chunk boobs, and tiny belly, because damn it, I was proud.

I was what my parents, grandparents, and other relatives called a "good eater."

And what kid doesn't want to be told they're good? Even if it is followed by the word *eater*.

What I didn't know at the time was that that was code for, "Cory's looking a little thick these days, maybe you should take away the Ding Dongs."

Instead, I thought, I am finally good at something. If I wasn't going to be great at ballet or tap or jazz like my little sister, and if I was always going to ride the bench in the park district's soccer leagues, at least I was going to be good at eating. In fact, I think there might have even been a point when I was striving to be great.

Some little girls fantasize about their weddings or growing up to be models, I just wanted to be a good eater.

And I would eat anything in sight, even if my tummy ached like no other—because I was determined to be recognized for my digestive skills.

Lucky for me, this newfound determination of mine arrived right before the summer my mom decided to open up an ice cream shop about ten minutes from our house. This was back in 1988 when frozen yogurt was all the rage. Remember TCBY, the predecessor to Pinkberry? This was a take on that. Only my mom's store served soft serve ice cream and Colombo frozen yogurt, with any toppings you wanted, plus hot dogs and chips. It was the Midwestern version of a healthy snack.

In other words, heaven for a fat kid like me.

I'm sure my sister and I were toted along to work that summer in an effort to teach us good work ethics and that a woman could do anything she wanted—even start her own business. But all I cared about was the free ice cream and the daily hot dog lunch, not the life lessons.

That summer, the Cone Shop became my home away from home, an Olympic training center for my sport.

At the time, we were living in Illinois in the same small town my parents had both grown up in, with many of my relatives still living nearby.

"Cory's a really good eater," my grandmother would say when we'd go over to her house for her famous spaghetti and meatballs.

I'd smile at her, take a bite of my dinner then finish my entire plate. Sometimes I'd ask for seconds and sometimes, though rarely, I'd just hold out for dessert. And usually she'd make sure to buy me my favorite—blueberry pie from

Bakers Square. Which I would then put in a bowl and mush up with vanilla ice cream until I basically had a soup of blueberries, crust, and melted dairy fat.

The thought of it repulses me now and makes me want to do 108 sun salutations, but back then it was my savior. The thing that kept me getting noticed and on track to being fantastic, the best eater ever.

Unfortunately, when I returned to school that fall, I realized there was a slight problem with my plan for greatness.

Because there's only so much you can eat in an effort to garner attention, before the kids at recess start to make fun of you and the life of the good eater begins to turn lonely.

I can still remember standing out on the blacktop playground next to my elementary school and being offered a piggyback ride, like little kids so often do with each other. But then my friend collapsed under my weight and I fell to the ground. The snickering of my schoolmates echoed all around. I coolly peeled myself from the asphalt and dusted off my behind as if nothing had happened, but inside I was mortified. Reality had set in. I wasn't a good eater, I was just fat.

For weeks, I tried to smile and laugh off the comments about my weight, but that only made things worse. A smile from a kid whose cheeks look like Chunk's from *The Goonies* always gets a laugh. But because I was such an introvert, I couldn't even redeem myself by being the funny fat kid, which made me realize that being a "good eater" wasn't so great after all.

However, I was a determined little kid, and the only reason I had gained that weight was to garner recognition, and I wasn't about to give up on my goals.

So it occurred to me that I needed something else to grab my classmates' attention.

If I was going to get noticed, I needed something bigger and better and with more bravado than finishing a giant hot dog in two minutes. I needed something spectacular. Something rare. Something no one could make fun of me for.

I needed...

CANCER.

And I needed it now.

But instead of wishing upon the stars or writing to Santa Claus, I knew if you really wanted something you had to pray to God. Or at least that's what all the priests and the teachers at CCD, the Catholic version of Sunday school, told me. So, I started praying for that cancer.

Now I lay me down to sleep, I pray the lord my soul to keep. And if I should get cancer before I wake, I'll thank the lord for heaven's sake.

I never wanted to die. Never even thought that was a possibility when I lay in my bed at nine years old and prayed to God that he would give me such a horrific disease.

Instead, I thought how cool it would be to get leukemia like the little girl, Wendy, who lived down the street. Everyone paid attention to her. The whole community showed their support, showering her family with gifts, love, and the all-important words, "what a strong little girl."

Wendy was ten years old. We had played some soccer together, but I really didn't know her. What I did know was that Wendy was this girl who everyone recognized for her strength and all I saw was that recognition.

Now, of course, I realize how hard and difficult it must have been for Wendy and her family to deal with the leukemia (and I pray today she is a healthy grown woman), but at nine years old all I heard was Wendy is so strong. And you, Cory, are a good eater.

Great, I had thought, I'm a good eater and the little leukemia girl is battling a life altering disease, why can't I have that instead? Why can't I be the one with the cool hats and the bald head, instead of the 100-pound fourth grader? Why can't people notice me? I can be strong. I can be cute in a hat. I can accept gifts graciously. But no, God or the universe or whoever else was in charge had different plans for me.

I was to be fat. Not prescribed chemotherapy.

Still, every night of my tenth year alive I prayed for cancer or any other disease that could bring the attention to me. I wanted my life to have meaning. I wanted to do something great. I wanted to be the poster child for some incurable disease.

I didn't want to be the shy kid with the elastic waistband pants.

I spent the next two years waiting to be struck with that cancer. I told God that if he gave me cancer he would see how strong I was and he would know that he'd made such a horrible mistake by giving any other kid the disease, because I would be the best patient yet. I would be the strongest cancer survivor ever.

Of course, I grew up, and we eventually moved to Indiana and by the time I got to high school, the weight of my childhood had seamlessly melted off, and I was perfectly healthy. I got busy being a teenager, and the prayer took a back burner to my life. As the boys started to take notice, I stopped the prayer completely. I had friends, boyfriends, and I actually turned out to be fairly athletic—I was a cheerleader who played varsity soccer and swam competitively.

In fact, I all but forgot about the prayer. That is, until May of 2007, when I first began this MS journey.

I remember the day when I first went to see the neurologist. It was a standard appointment to follow up on the numbness that I had told my regular doctor about. She proceeded with a neurological exam, took down my symptoms, and checked my reflexes. At that point, she wasn't sure what I had and that was when the other possibilities were thrown out there. She asked if I had ever had migraines. I said no. Then she asked if I knew what Lyme disease was. I said yes, the hot older cousin of my friend Amy had it (of course I left out the hot part); I knew that you got it from tick bites and I knew that it could leave you incredibly sick and weak for years.

The neurologist said she'd have to run some more tests. I said fine, but I never remembered getting bit by a tick. In fact, my sister and I spent so much time in the woods behind our house when we were growing up, that looking for ticks when you returned from playing outside was just as much a part of our routine as it was to take off our shoes when we came inside.

I allowed the doctor to draw blood and I returned home that night in shock. Something was actually wrong with me. How had this happened?

And then, I remembered... *Dear God, It's me, Cory, please give me cancer.*

Upon remembering the prayer, I immediately dropped onto my bed and began to sob. Praying like I'd never prayed before...

God, I was young and naïve. I was lonely and an outsider and I just wanted people to notice me. I wasn't serious. Okay, maybe I was then, but that was 19 years ago. Things are different now. I don't need cancer to show how strong I am. In fact, I don't even want to be strong. I'm okay with admitting I need help. I've learned that lesson. God, please, I don't need the attention. I don't even want it. I don't want people to look at me and feel sorry. I like who am. I love who I am. Please don't mess with my life.

That night, I cried myself to sleep. I couldn't believe my prayer was coming true. Okay, so it wasn't cancer, but it was something, and I cursed, "Who in their right mind wants to be sick?" Apparently, a lonely nine-year-old.

The next morning I woke up feeling a little bit better. I had no new test results, and no definitive answers, maybe my neurologist was just being cautious.

Of course, I now know that to be false, that they've narrowed down the possibilities and the only explanation they can give for my symptoms and the spots on my brain is MS, but at least I don't have cancer and maybe God has forgotten the prayer.

But now it's February 2008. It's been eight months since that first appointment with the neurologist and I am sitting in the MS specialist's office waiting to get the results of a spinal MRI. The evoked potential tests had come back negative and the specialist had ordered a scan of my back to see if there are any lesions on my spinal cord.

The room is full of MS patients at various stages of the disease. There's a man with a cane. A woman in a wheelchair. A lady with a walker. And several others who, like me, look perfectly healthy, but probably suffer from invisible symptoms.

After staring at the wall and reading magazines in the waiting room, the nurse finally calls me back to one of the exam rooms.

I am, once again, alone at another doctor's appointment. My parents haven't flown out this time, because at this point, what more could the doctor say? Yes, you now definitely have MS. And I didn't ask Randy to come with me, because besides telling him about the disease that one night in bed, I haven't brought it up since.

So, I'm sitting in the cold plastic chair waiting for the specialist, when she walks in with a smile on her face.

"How've you been feeling?" she asks.

I tell her that besides the pins and needles sensations and the pain that keeps me up at night and all of the other subtle symptoms, like my damn memory loss, and inability to find the right words nothing has really changed since the last time I saw her in December.

"That's good to hear," she says. "Well, I have some other good news. Your tests came back normal. There are no lesions on your spine."

"So, what does that mean?" I ask, hoping she'll say she made a horrible mistake and I don't actually have MS. That God may have finally heard my prayer: *I don't want to be sick.*

"Well, I still believe in my heart that you have MS and at some point it will reveal itself on one of these tests."

I am thrown by her choice of words. People are supposed to "believe in their hearts" that love is beautiful and one day I'll find my prince, or that everything's going to be okay. Not that I have an incurable disease. "Now what?" I ask, wondering why she can't just tell me that I absolutely have the disease and I should start taking the disease modifying drugs right away.

"We can do one of two things. We can wait until June and you can have another brain MRI, because it will have been over six months from your last one. And we can see if any more lesions have developed. If they have, we'll have a definitive diagnosis. If not, then we'll need to wait some more and see."

Before she can continue, I ask, "So there's nothing we can do for a more clear answer?" I didn't want to wait in limbo land any longer, wanted instead to be told "yes" or "no," not "most likely."

"Well, we can do a spinal tap in a week or so."

I gasp in horror. "What will that do?"

She tells me that a large percentage of patients with MS have what they call oligoclonal bands in their spinal fluid. Unfortunately, not everyone who has MS has them.

"So, what you're saying is I can let you tap my spine or I can get an MRI in six months and there's still a possibility that these will both come back negative, but you'll still tell me you believe I have MS?"

"That's correct."

"And is there a time when you'll tell me I don't have MS? Like how many more tests with no progression do I need to have?"

"I really think we need to keep testing you for a while."

I contemplate my options: wait another six months or have a giant needle stuck in my spine.

"The spinal tap really isn't that bad, and it can be very telling," she says, trying to ease my apprehension, but not doing much to quell my fears.

"You know what? I think I'll wait," I finally say. There's no way in hell I'm going to allow her to do the spinal tap, especially if it's not going to tell me with 100 percent certainty whether I have MS or not.

"That's fine," she says as she writes up the order for the brain MRI. "I'll see you in six months then."

I start to gather up my stuff to leave, but all of a sudden she puts out her hand and stops me.

"There's something else I need to go over with you."

Something else? What else could there be? If she tells me she has one other crazy test option that only gives inconclusive results, I'm running.

"When they did your spinal MRI they saw some lesions on your thyroid."

I slouch back into my chair. That doesn't sound good.

"What kind of lesions?" I ask.

"Actually, they're cysts."

"Okay, so?" I ask, hoping it means nothing.

"You should probably see your regular doctor and have her take a further look. But I'm going to order you an ultrasound and then you can follow up with her for the results."

I am in utter shock. How did this convo go from lesions on the brain to mass uncertainty to now I have to have my thyroid investigated?

"I'm sure it's nothing," she says, "but it's better to have it looked at just in case."

"In case what?" I ask.

"You should get the ultrasound, then talk to your regular doctor. She should be able to answer your questions."

"Fine. Is there anything else?" I ask out of frustration, hoping to God there really isn't anything else.

"That's it. I'll see you in June." And with that she leaves me alone with a stack of papers: An order for a brain MRI, and an order for a thyroid ultrasound.

I then gather up all my stuff and head out the door. Two words ingrained in my head:

Thyroid. Cysts.

Of course, as soon as I arrive home I Google that shit and find three answers to my new problem.

One: I could have Hashimoto's, which is a thyroid disease that my mom actually has and is fairly manageable.

Two: it could be totally benign. And…

Three: I could have cancer.

MOTHERFUCKER!

I look up and fold my hands together, *Are you serious, God? Really? We're back to this again? Will I ever live down that prayer?*

I close the Safari browser window on my Mac laptop and open up my calendar so that I can call the ultrasound center and schedule my appointment. But when I see that today is Fat Tuesday, I stop myself from reaching for the phone. I take a deep breath and think, perhaps it's a sign I should start following my faith again and give something up for Lent.

Then I give it some thought…

But seeing how I'm not having sex, and I don't smoke, nor eat crappy food—the things I would normally give up—I decide to give up the thing that's causing the most pain and chaos in my life.

Doctors.

If I can avoid them for 40 days then at least no one can give me any more bad news and if I can obey the rules of Catholicism, even if it has been years since I've set foot in a church, maybe everything will be all right.

I put the ultrasound order in the top drawer of my desk then I fold my hands and make my pledge…

I'm giving up doctors for Lent.

Then I pray…

Now I lay me down to sleep, I pray the lord my soul to keep. And if I say please, will you stop threatening me with disease? Please!

Then I unfold my hands and make the sign of the cross over my heart...

Because, Lord knows, if there were ever a time I needed God on my side it's now.

Chapter Sixteen

WALK OF SHAME

I t's official. I am going to hell.

Bless me father, for I have sinned, it has been at least ten years since my last confession if not more and, if I can be frank, I've sort of been a whore.

Well, not exactly a whore, but I'm pretty sure that having sex with an ex-lover, while dating a new man, who you have yet to sleep with, isn't exactly Madonna territory.

Yes, Randy and I are still dating. No, we have not done the deed. And it is now mid-March, only a week from Easter.

So, while I have managed to avoid doctors for some 30-odd days, I haven't exactly been able to keep "it" out of my pants. Some women would argue that I've done nothing wrong. I'd already slept with Brad plenty of times in the past. Randy and I never talked about any exclusivity in our relationship, and I didn't even give up sex for Lent.

But I still can't help feeling like I've crossed some sort of Pope-drawn line, because when I wake up that Sunday morning, curled up in Brad's bed, the first voice I hear isn't his, but his mother's.

"Brad, do you want to come upstairs for breakfast?" her soft voice echoes over the intercom, so quietly at first that I think perhaps I am dreaming.

Only, when I open my eyes and see Brad's naked behind peeping out of the covers, it occurs to me that this situation is all too real.

I am at Brad's place, sure, but he had recently been kicked out of his apartment because the landlord had sold the place to a developer, so he is temporarily living in his parents' guest quarters. I say *quarters* and not *house* because while the place has its own full bathroom, kitchen, and side door entrance, it is technically still a part of the main house, a main house that, I might add, is quite a mansion. Complete with pool, Jacuzzi, tennis courts, and breathtaking views of the Pacific Ocean.

So when Brad, an ex I'd converted into a friend, called me that Saturday evening to invite me over to catch up and hang out in the Jacuzzi, I had no problem accepting the offer. I figured it'd be nice to see a familiar face, that I would go over there for a couple of hours, we'd chat like old friends, and then I would come home for a good night's rest.

Well, two bottles of wine later, that theory went out the door and before I knew it, I was pouring my heart out to Brad about the possible cancer in my throat, my fears about the MS, and the fact that I worried no one would ever find me attractive again. This led to a hug of consolation, which led to 45 minutes in the Jacuzzi, which led to a confession that he still thought I was hot, which led to several long passionate kisses, which led to my sin in the bedroom, which leads us to…

"Brad! Are you up? We made pancakes."

I quickly pull the covers tight against me. Like I said, this is one of those fancy houses: If his mom can intercom us, who knows what she can see?

Brad finally opens his eyes and smiles. Then he whispers to me.

"Do you want pancakes?"

"Seriously?" I ask, pulling the covers tighter.

"Yeah, why not?"

"Um, because, it's seven-thirty in the morning and I'm quite certain that your parents aren't going to think I just stopped by a few minutes ago."

"So, I'll tell them you spent the night."

"No, don't. Can't I sneak out this door and leave so they'll never know I was here?"

I start to get up. I can see my jeans and shirt sitting on the chair across the room, but Brad stops me.

"Come on, they won't care. They like you."

"They met me once. And that time I didn't just sleep with their son," I reply as I stare at my clothes, hoping I could move them onto my body with the force of my mind.

"Brad. You better get up soon. Your father has to go to the office and I need you to drive me to church."

I look at Brad, *please don't.*

"I'll be right there. Is it okay if Cory comes too? We had some wine last night, so she stayed over," he shouts out to the intercom on the wall.

I pick up my pillow and start hitting Brad. *You dumbass!*

"Sure, that's fine, I'll have your dad make some extra bacon. See you in a few," she says then clicks off.

"Are you serious? I can't go up there. What am I going to say? Oh, yeah, I got drunk last night, banged your son, and didn't feel like driving home, so I hope you don't mind if I join you for a nice family breakfast."

"Seriously, it's going to be fine. They know you're

my friend. And besides, I'm an adult, what can they say anyway?"

"That your friend Cory is a whore."

"I suppose they could. But I doubt they will. They're a little too conservative for that."

"Thanks. That makes me feel a whole lot better."

So, while Brad gets to put on a fresh pair of clothes, I re-dress myself in the exact same outfit I was wearing the night before, skinny jeans and a long-sleeved black T-shirt. I use some Kleenex to wipe off the mascara and eyeliner that had shifted from its rightful place in the heat of last night and try to look somewhat presentable. But really? I look like hell.

And I am about to take the longest walk of shame in my life.

After the five-minute walk up the stairs, down the side corridor, around the game room, past a guest bedroom, through the parlor, and into the kitchen, I timidly say, "Good morning."

Mrs. Mom of Brad immediately warms up to me and offers juice and coffee. I politely decline the coffee, as I don't drink caffeine, and graciously take the orange juice.

"Can I help you with anything?" I ask, silently thanking my mom for the etiquette classes in Chicago she dragged me to on a weekly basis when I was 11.

"No, no. Have a seat," Brad's mom says as she points to a chair at the table.

"Thanks," I say as I make my way over to the solid mahogany kitchen table, trying my best to smile at Mr. Dad of Brad and play innocent, but I know he can tell I am not a good Catholic girl who had just had a few too many sips of wine the night before.

"Pancakes are ready. Brad, can you grab the bacon," he says without even a glance my way.

As Brad grabs the bacon and heads over to the table where I have now taken a seat, I give him one of those all telling looks: *I can't believe you dragged me up here.*

But Brad just shrugs his shoulders with a smile and takes the seat opposite my own.

His mom sits to my left and his father quietly takes a seat on my right.

As much as I'm enjoying the fact that I get to indulge in a wonderful breakfast feast, complete with pancakes, bacon, and fresh OJ, I'm still sitting on the edge of my chair waiting for one of the parental units to start harassing me about the fact that I just shacked in their guest quarters with their baby son.

If the situation were the other way around, and Brad had just spent the night at my parents' place, my mom would have already fired a round of a hundred questions and poor Brad would probably have to think of a million and one ways to explain the fact that he slept in my bed. But my mom is not dumb and usually calls a guy out on his intentions. Like the summer after my junior year in college when I went back home to Indiana for a month and dated this guy, Craig. We liked to go camping in Michigan a lot because it was fun and rustic and a little romantic, but one night as I was saying bye to my mom before we headed out, she totally called us out on the situation.

"What's the difference between camping and getting a hotel room? I know what you two are going to go do."

Craig stood there speechless, for he knew he'd been found out, but I quickly covered. "Camping's different. We get to make a fire and have s'mores. It's more fun. And we're not doing what you think we are."

"Fine, but just be safe," she said as she sent us on our way with a smirk.

Craig was mortified and couldn't believe my mom had been so blunt. But I was used to this kind of openness and shrugged it off, much in the same way Brad is doing right now.

Which is why I think I am so petrified that someone is going to say something. I'm used to mothers being brutally honest, so if Brad's mom is anything like mine, she's bound to say something like...

"I heard..." Oh my God, I think. Here it comes. She's going to tell us that she heard everything last night. The creaky bed, the sighs of pleasure... But then she finishes her sentence. "I heard you're writing a book."

"Yeah," I respond with a sigh of relief.

"That's great," she says. "Brad told me about everything you've been going through. I'm so sorry."

"Thanks," I say with reserve. It's the only thing I know how to say. I don't really like talking about the MS to people. I'm afraid I might freak them out, that I'll say something that might make them not want to talk to me again. Luckily, Brad interjects before his mom has a chance to say anymore.

"I'm going to do a 150-mile bike ride with Cory in October," he says.

"Really?" she asks.

"He is. It's a charity event to raise money for MS research," I say proudly. Because this is the type of thing people want to hear. They want to hear how you're overcoming the odds or facing a disabling disease head on by training your body to do things most unaffected people wouldn't even dream of doing.

"Do you think you're in shape for that?" Brad's dad asks him. The first words that have really come out of his mouth the entire morning.

"I've got some time," Brad laughs then turns to me, "we should start bike riding together."

"Sure," I say, then add to his dad, "My parents are going to do the ride too. So, I'm hoping if they can do it, so can Brad."

"That's wonderful," his mom adds. "Where do you ride from?"

"It starts in Irvine and you ride along the coast down to San Diego with an overnight stay in Carlsbad."

"Brad, you should book a hotel room for then, right?" his dad asks in a tone that says you better have your own room, because I don't want to hear about you slumbering with Cory again.

"Um, yeah," Brad says. "I guess so."

"Good," his dad says with a nod before he turns to me. "And as for you ..." he starts and I think, here it is. My punishment for shacking at the house. For having slept with their son. For taking a walk of shame past their antique grand piano. "You know that if you ever need anything you're always welcome over here. Any time."

"Thanks," I respond with a smile. Then think ...

Maybe the walk of shame isn't the worst thing to ever happen to a girl. Maybe the walk of shame is there to serve as a reminder that you are not alone in this fight against the world. That you can walk with someone else in the war against this invisible disease, even if it is with the dad of the guy you just committed a carnal sin with.

Chapter Seventeen

MILF

My mom is a total MILF.

And she is probably going to kill me for writing that, but it's the truth.

She is hot.

Obviously, this isn't something I came up with on my own. It was a declaration that came about when I was in high school. The year was 1997, I was 17 and my mom was all of 38 years old. She was cool, well dressed, and pretty. Also, she was once Homecoming Queen, which is why my prom date senior year and his friends all liked to joke about how my mom was a "Mom I'd Like to F…" okay, I think you know the rest.

The only reason this is important is because I am essentially my mother's twin, and I am secretly hoping that when I grow up, or, more appropriately, get knocked up, I too will be a MILF.

Apparently, these are the kinds of aspirations that go through one's mind when one is waiting to have one's body scanned to look for cancerous growths. Because these are the thoughts running over and over in my head as I sit here waiting for my thyroid ultrasound.

Easter has passed, Lent is over, and according to my Catholic upbringing, I am finally allowed to see the doctors again. I'm at the UCLA facility in Santa Monica, sitting in the ultrasound waiting room preparing to have those cysts on my thyroid scanned and photographed as if they were my own little children.

There's a moderate-sized fish tank in the back of the small room and the walls are that obligatory putty color that seems to be in every medical waiting room I've been in over the past seven months. The place is pretty packed with patients and everyone either has a smile on their face or a man by their side. Because, besides me and some woman who looks to be about 65, every other woman in here is fully preggers.

I look over at one of the expectant moms and her cute husband and smile. I think about what an adorable family they're going to have and wonder if it's a boy or a girl. I'm about to make small talk and congratulate the young couple, when the mom-to-be shoots me the most lethal look: *Back off, bitch.* I am completely taken aback. Shouldn't this be a friendly office? A waiting room full of good news? *It's a girl. You're having a boy. Can you hear the heartbeat? There're her fingernails.* But this woman is not happy. I smile again, this time catching the eye of her husband, who smiles back at me. At least someone's in a good mood. But his smile only makes the daggers shooting out of the woman's eyes pierce deeper into my skin.

I quickly grab one of the baby magazines on the chair next to me so as not to continue to accidentally catch her eye, or that of her man. I flip through the magazine trying to look for an article that might actually apply to me, but let's face it, I read *Glamour* and articles about how to please my man in bed, not how to get my newborn baby boy to go to bed.

I pretend to be interested in the magazine and try to go unnoticed when my stomach gives a little rumble and I instinctively reach for it. I watch as another mom looks over at me with a sympathetic smile and as I do, it suddenly occurs to me, the dagger lady must think I'm here to have my baby's first photograph taken. She thinks I'm pregnant too and considering the fact that I am here all alone, I must appear pretty pathetic and desperate. No wonder she doesn't want me looking at her husband.

I probably look like some damsel in distress who is searching for a man to step in, be her baby's daddy, and whisk her away to safety and security.

Out of nervousness, I start to twist the silver Tiffany ring on my right hand. For a moment, I contemplate doing the switcheroo—taking the ring and placing it on my left hand, a trick I've learned over the years as I've frequented many bars where some not-so-suitable suitors have approached me. Under the table I'd do the switch, then hold up my left hand with a smile and say, "Sorry, I'm married," and they usually get the hint and walk away. But I'm guessing that the mom-to-be who just gave me the death stare will probably notice my trick and not really think it's funny right now.

I contemplate telling the mom the truth of my situation.

You see, Mrs. Pregnant Lady with Cute Husband, I am pretty independent and don't normally need a man, but when my neurologist told me I had this incurable, potentially debilitating disease, all I could think about was who the heck is going to want to marry me now, and so, here I am single, and dating, however, the guy I'm currently seeing still won't have sex with me, so no, I'm not actually knocked up, unless of course, I am carrying the next baby Jesus, which might be a nice twist to the story and force God to look down upon me with some mercy for once and possibly make the potential cancer that's growing on my thyroid disappear, but beyond that I'm just waiting here alone to have an ultrasound of my throat, so if you could lay off the dirty looks I would greatly appreciate it while I consider the fact that on top of my other disease I may have cancer too.

But, obviously, I can't say this out loud. Those daggers she shot earlier would certainly turn into piercing icicles. And, let's be honest, I'm kind of a quiet person.

Confront someone face to face? Not my style. But write a letter and place it on some bitchy woman's car windshield when she yells at you in the parking lot of your favorite sandwich place? Now, that I have done.

It was this past Christmas season. I had only been sitting with the news of the MS for about two months and was in the beginning stages of dating Randy. On this particular day I was in a pretty healthy emotional place. I hadn't cried in weeks and I had begun to feel semi-normal again. Or so I thought.

I was waiting in the extremely crowded parking lot of Bay Cities Deli in Santa Monica. Randy and a bunch of my friends and their significant others were coming over for a holiday dinner later that night and I was picking up some of the deli's famous bread and a couple of appetizers.

I usually avoid this deli on weekends and during peak lunch hours, as the small parking lot only holds 20 or so cars and it tends to turn into a madhouse, but it was late on a Friday afternoon and I figured it wouldn't be so bad. What I failed to take into account was the fact that this was the holiday season and I probably wasn't the only one hosting a festive dinner.

When I finally pulled off the street and into the lot, the security guard/parking attendant motioned for me to drive forward and wait for a spot ahead. After I inched forward a bit, I put my car in park and waited out of the way of traffic.

I turned on the radio and started jamming to the Christmas tune recorded by 'NSync, "Merry Christmas, and happy holidays…" I was patiently waiting for my turn to park and in no rush. It was the holiday season and I saw no point in getting my panties in a bunch over something as simple as having to wait to park my car.

Unfortunately, the woman behind me missed the memo on patience and had it in her head that this waiting thing was completely below her.

She rolled down her window and screamed out, "What the hell are you doing? Move it!"

I came out of my Christmas carol daze and looked up at her with a smile and politely motioned that I was waiting for the next spot to open.

This was obviously not the kind of response she wanted from me, because she immediately swerved around to the side of my Jeep, hit the gas, and started screaming obscenities at me as she raced into one of the two hidden spots behind the deli that had just opened, and which I had failed to notice.

"Are you an idiot? Why the hell would you wait there?!" she continued to scream as she got out of her parked car and I pulled into the other spot, which was right next to hers. I stayed inside my car and rolled down the window a few inches, as she continued to tell me how ridiculous I was for waiting and how pissed she was that I had held her up.

My only retort was, "It's the holidays, be nice."

She responded with another dirty look, screamed, "Bitch!," slammed her car door, and headed inside the store.

Before I could come up with some smart response, all the stress of the MS, the constant doctor's appointments, and the constant wondering of what was going to happen next, came crashing down all around me. Pair that with the woman's hostility and my eyes burst into an immediate hailstorm of tears. My body began shaking and I went into full uncontrollable sobbing mode. For five minutes I let this continue, snot and all.

I was a mess, but eventually I managed to calm myself down and pull it together. I wiped the salty tears from my cheeks and applied a fresh coat of shiny red lip gloss. I glanced in the rear view mirror. I didn't look perfect, but I was presentable so I got out of my car and made my way inside.

I went to the back of the deli, grabbed a couple loaves of bread and some fancy cheese and headed for the sandwich area.

When I had originally left my house, I had big ambitions to also grab a "small turkey with the works no mayo mild peppers muenster cheese" for a late lunch after I got what I needed for the dinner I was preparing, but when I passed by the crazed parking lot lady who was also waiting in the sandwich line and she started glaring at me again, my hands immediately clenched and my bottom lip started to tremble.

Don't cry. Don't cry. I told myself over and over.

I couldn't let this woman see me fall apart. So instead of grabbing a number for a sandwich, I took my stuff and headed for the cash register.

As I left the store, I thought I would break down again, but something strange happened. An extreme feeling of strength came over me.

After all the medical shit I'd been dealing with, this lady's rudeness didn't even compare, so instead of getting into my car and racing out of the parking lot, I grabbed a scrap piece of paper from my backseat and I started to write.

Dear Miss,

Next time you decide to use unkind words, please think twice and understand that you may not know someone's life situation. I was recently diagnosed with MS and am still in shock from the news. Please know that while I held back my tears, I said a silent prayer wishing you and your family all the love and joy in the world during this holiday season!!!

I read it over several times to ensure the passive-aggressive message was clear, then I got out of my car, placed the note on the woman's windshield and left the parking lot with my hands still shaking, fearful that this woman would come after me and call me a bitch once again.

Two blocks down the road, I called my sister, who was living in North Carolina for grad school, and burst into tears. Only this time it was a cry of relief. I told her what I had done and she said she was proud of me and couldn't believe that her shy older sister had done something so bold.

And when everyone came over that night for my holiday dinner I was in the best mood.

The kind of mood that I'm trying to re-create as I sit here in the waiting room of the ultrasound place. Because I need that strength to bring me out of this funk.

The funk of a single girl in a room full of mothers-to-be and their happy husbands, dodging dirty looks.

When the death stare woman and her husband are finally called away, I start to take a few precautionary measures, lest another woman and her cute betrothed arrive and they too decide I'm lusting after the Y chromosome half of their twosome. First, I try to stick out my gut a bit, hoping to transform the tuna salad sandwich I had for lunch into a baby bump. Then I grab a baby magazine and pretend to be interested. And I am about to move my ring over to my other hand when I am suddenly called back by a nurse.

She brings me to a small dark room and hands me a hospital issue top to put on instead of the shirt I'm wearing. As I change, I thank God that I wore my pretty bra just in case the ultrasound technician happens to be a hot guy.

But it's not. It's just some woman who looks to be only a few years older than myself. She tells me to lay down on the bed then puts that jelly stuff all over my throat.

"This might be a bit cold," she says. "But it should warm up once I get going."

"That's fine," I say as she turns on the machine and starts to rub the little sensor thing on my neck. I wait for her to turn the screen towards me like they do in the movies when they're showing the moms their babies, but the woman keeps the screen angled so that only she can see it.

"Ummm," I start to say, but by the look on the technician's face and her sealed lips I know she doesn't want me to talk.

"I need you to stay still," she says.

"Okay," I say.

"And quiet too."

I shut my mouth and try to arch my neck so that I can see the little guys that are growing on my thyroid. But the woman presses more firmly on my skin with the sensor and I go back to staring at the ceiling.

I start to think how this isn't fair. It's my body. I should be entitled to see what's going on inside it. But noooo....

There's a rule: When there's a baby growing inside you, they're all too happy to show you every bit of the image, but when there's a possible tumor, they angle that machine so it's impossible to see the screen.

This rule of secrecy does nothing to raise my happiness level and I start to come up with scenarios about what the images on the screen look like.

Are the cysts blobs? Or big dark spots on an otherwise healthy organ? I wonder if they look like tiny babies. Oooh, and how many are there? What if I'm having septuplets? Seven nodules of dangerous tissue growing inside me.

Maybe I can have my own show on TLC.

Cory plus seven equals... PENIS!

What? But then I realize I've overheard the conversation in the next room.

Muffled voices are coming through the wall behind my head. While most of what's being said is quite distorted I can make out a happy mother and the father to be oohing and ahhing over what must be the image of their tiny little baby. A baby they've been informed is a boy. It must be one of the most exciting moments in their lives. A small smile starts to form on my face but when my lips move the technician presses at my throat a little harder.

Damn you, lady, this is not fun for me either. Can't I just see them for a second? I want to see my little pieces of cancer. I want to call out to the universe, *Hello, my little cancer babies… where are your feet? I don't hear your heartbeat, maybe you're dead, or even better, maybe you don't exist.*

Because, really, if I can see those things maybe I can will them away. Maybe I can will it all away.

Then a thought crosses my mind, *What if I don't have MS at all, what if all these weird symptoms have been caused by thyroid cancer and all my worrying about the MS will have been for naught? What if my MILF dreams do come true? What if all I have is a* Malignance *I have to* Learn to Fight? *What if that's it? What if I'm just a Leo living with cancer, not a Ms. with MS?*

The woman finishes the scan then leaves me to get dressed. As soon as I sit up, I promptly look over at the screen, but she's already turned the machine off.

I sigh in defeat.

There will be no souvenir photos of the babies in my throat, only a week of waiting to determine the sex—benign or cancer.

Chapter Eighteen

PLAN B

I 'm over celebrities and velvet ropes, I just want to
get laid.

Disrobe. Screw. Repeat. That is my plan.

At 25, a trip to Vegas looked like this:

Fly in from LA on a Friday night. Meet up with your
publicist friends at the Hard Rock. Get slapped with several wristbands to get you VIP access for that night's event.
Run into your old boss. Get in the limo with him and his
entourage. Head to Caesars. Get special treatment at the
Pussycat Dolls Lounge because you're now sitting at a table
with its creator, Robin Antin. Go back to the Hard Rock.
Have Brent Bolthouse flag your crew into Body English
past the swarms of people waiting to get inside. Find your
friends. Dance next to No Doubt's table. Have the drummer
offer you a drink. Sip Vodka Red Bull as you listen to Velvet
Revolver. Shut the place down. Dance with Tone Lōc, the
late-'80s rapper. Hit the craps table when your friend gets
called back to work to find a private jet so Jessica Simpson
can get home. Win several hundred bucks. Call it a night
when you can see the sun rising outside the glass doors of
the casino. Jump into the elevator. Get pushed to the back
as Jeremy Piven slams a buxom blonde up against the mirrored wall next to you. Open the door to your room. Crash
on the bed in your clothes from the night before. Sleep for

five hours. Wake up. Go to the pool. Hang with a bachelor party. Drink some more. Eat some food. Stay out all night. Pass out again.

That's how I used to roll.

This time around, however, I'm looking to do a little more than eat, sleep, repeat. At 28, I've got a bigger, more sophisticated plan.

S. E. X.

But don't think I'm about to let loose my dark side and sleep with a man I barely know in Vegas. I have standards and rules. One of which is no sleeping with strangers while in the state of Nevada. I say Nevada because I've had one or two slipups with some unknowns in California and, well, that state is my home, so it's safe. But Vegas? You can't do that there. That city is like a box of chocolates, you never know what you're going to get.

So, no, I have never slept with anyone in Vegas, stranger or not, which is why this trip is going to be different.

For the first time ever I am going to Vegas with a man I am seeing. A man I have yet to sleep with and a man I have every intention of stripping down naked and making love to.

I am going with Randy and this is going to be a romantic trip.

It's May of 2008. Randy's just finished law school and is about to start studying for the bar, so we figured this would be a nice weekend to get away before he's completely consumed by the law. Personally, I'm kind of hoping we can break a few laws. Or at least commit a few carnal sins. I haven't gotten the results back from my thyroid ultrasound and I never told him about the procedure. He already knows about the MS. Why worry him with other minor details? Besides, this trip is about much more. Like connecting, getting closer, furthering our relationship, and, you know, sex. Unfortunately, Randy has other ideas. More civilized ideas—like gambling, drinking, getting dressed up, and going to nice dinners.

Which is great. I love dinner at Lawry's. Throwing money down at the craps table, betting on roulette together, lying out by the pool, drinking cocktails at the Wynn. Those are all fun things to do when you're on a two-day getaway with the man you're really into, but sex? Well, that's a different story.

As you know, Randy and I have had some difficulties in that department.

His rules on nakedness, i.e., if my top's off, his must stay on, coupled with the fact that I've been going through the "I hate my body because of this disease" phase, and we don't normally get too far in the bedroom.

But Vegas is supposed to be different.

Not that I've iterated any of this to Randy, but he's a guy and I'm assuming that since he invited me to Vegas to stay in a hotel room with him for two nights this is exactly what's been on his mind as well. Perhaps the fact that we haven't slept together has nothing to do with my self-loathing and his prudishness and only to do with the fact that he wants our first time to be special and that's where Vegas comes into play.

When we finally check into our modern rock and roll inspired room at the Hard Rock and put down our bags I think this might be it.

He looks at me with his big blue eyes then says, "Come here."

I move to him. He pulls me close then runs his hands through my hair and gently guides me to the bed where my knees buckle and I collapse into the fluffy white down comforter. He falls on top of me and we continue to kiss and caress each other with passion. After a while his hand begins to make its way up to second base and I start to think we're going to keep going as he touches my bare skin. But just as his cold fingers send shivers down my spine, he pulls away and stops himself.

"It's already four o'clock. We should go see the old part of Vegas now before it gets dark."

"Okay," I reply as I sit up and straighten my shirt. I guess he must have bigger plans for our first time. I slip on my shoes and apply a fresh coat of lip gloss and smooth my hair.

We head out to the downtown area of the city and arrive at one of the original casinos where I imagine my grandparents used to gamble, back in the day when they'd fly out here to watch Ol' Blue Eyes perform.

"Do you know how to play craps?" he asks.

"Yeah, I do, but it's been a while, so you'll have to help me," I say in my best helpless girl voice, not wanting to let on to the fact that the last time I played craps was with my dad who taught me all the tricks of the trade and I ended up winning enough money to pay my rent for a month and buy a four-carat blue topaz David Yurman ring. However, I know better than to tell him all these details. After my sister once told my grandma how she beat her boyfriend at golf, my grandma was mortified and advised her not to beat a boy again or they'll never want to be with you. Ever since then, I've known not to brag about my skills, especially if I was trying to seal the deal.

So I let Randy tell me when to "press the six," and bet the "horn high yo" and we make enough money to pay for dinner that night.

After dinner we gamble some more and sip on cocktails until finally the clock strikes three and we decide to head to bed. I slip out of my dress in the privacy of the bathroom, and put on a pair of shorts and a tank top. I get into bed and wait as Randy brushes his teeth and puts on his own pajamas. In hindsight, I probably should've packed something smaller and lacier to sleep in, but as much as I want to make love to Randy, there is still a part of me that is scared out of my mind.

I haven't had sex in what seems like forever and I worry that I am not going to know what to do, or it'll be awkward, or something embarrassing will happen. I'm also sure there's a small part of me that's hoping if I don't dress too sexy then I won't have to actually go through with my plan of getting laid.

But Randy soon comes back to bed and for the first time ever in our relationship we both have our shirts off. It's exhilarating and fun and after some time, my shorts are gone too and as my panties begin to slip off, I ask, "Do you have a condom?"

"Um, actually, no..."

We stop right there in our nakedness and I pause in thought. Had he not planned for this? Does he not want to do this? I know I was the one with the plan, but I was convinced he'd want this too. Now I am embarrassed. What if he doesn't even want to have sex with me?

"Sorry, I forgot to pack them," he says.

"Oh," I say, a little bit relieved because at least he'd thought about it.

"I know exactly where they are next to my bed at home, if that helps."

"Well, I'm not on the pill," I say with a pang of disappointment as I silently curse my body. Why can't I tolerate the pill like most other women? Why does sex have to be so complicated? First it's the MS, now it's my inability to be on birth control.

"I guess we should just sto—," he starts. *He really doesn't want me, does he*? I have to think of something.

"Wait!" I shout before he can say any more. "This is Vegas. Check the minibar, I bet they have them there."

Randy immediately jumps at the idea and gets out of bed. But when he gets to the minibar his testosterone fueled search takes a strange turn.

"There's a can of nuts for 11 dollars, a bottle of water for five. Can you believe these prices? Oh, but they have M&Ms. Do you like peanut or plain better? They have vodka too and a cigar, and three types of Gatorade, a razor blade, a Payday bar…" He continues to read off and comment upon every item on the list. With each word he mutters the bulge in his pants gets smaller and smaller. Finally, he gets to the end, "uh, I don't see any condoms."

"Are you sure?" I ask with one last ounce of hope, even though I know the moment is over and he's literally just filibustered his way out of having sex with me by standing up there and reading off the entire contents of the minibar.

"Yeah," he says as he retreats to the bed. "Should we go to sleep? Maybe try again tomorrow?"

"Sure," I say, then say no more. I don't want to be the girl who has to beg for sex. I put on my shorts in silence. I don't know what else to say. Am I supposed to get mad at him for not having condoms? For not wanting to do me? It's not like he threw shit at me, or verbally assaulted me. Has he really done anything wrong?

The next morning, Randy wakes me with a tap on the shoulder.

"Good morning," I reply and lean over to kiss him, with the hope that maybe last night was all a dream, and I hadn't been rejected by the lack of latex, but his lack of affection makes me realize it was all too real. He quickly kisses my cheek then hops out of bed and throws on a pair of jeans.

"It's already eleven, let's get up and walk around the strip. Maybe see if we can get tickets to *Love*. You can shower first. I'm going to run downstairs and get some bottled water so it doesn't cost a fortune. Do you want anything?"

Well, I could name one thing, but I don't say the word. He'd offered to go to the store so maybe he is already thinking the same thing.

"Uh, maybe a juice or something would be nice and whatever else you think we might need," I say, hoping he gets the hint and buys some Trojans.

After he returns and we finish getting ready, we spend the day exploring the strip. We play some roulette, find out that Cirque du Soleil's *Love* is sold out, and sip mai tais at the Trader Vic's that has just opened.

All in all, it's a great day, full of conversation and laughter, but there is no mention of sex, or lack thereof, so I figure Randy has things under control. That he bought condoms earlier and later that night we'll enjoy our first time together in romantic bliss. I think I can just keep quiet and not say a thing. After all, isn't that the town slogan? *What happens in Vegas, stays in Vegas?*

Unfortunately, that line doesn't really apply when you're actually in Vegas, because I should've said something to Randy. I should've brought up the awkward situation of the night before and made sure that he'd bought the prophylactics.

That night, after dinner, drinks, and gambling until five a.m., Randy and I are once again in bed together, only this time we are both fully undressed. I think that this is it. That the big moment has finally come. That I have hit the jackpot, and I am going to collect my prize.

But just as he goes to stick his coin into my penny slot, he pulls away and stops.

"We can't do this," he says.

Oh great, here comes the truth. He hates me. He hates sex. He hates me and sex.

"Why?" I ask.

"We don't have any condoms."

"What?" Now I am pissed.

"I forgot."

"I thought that's why you went to the store earlier."

He stutters for a second and I think about what to do. I could just let him off the hook, turn over and go to sleep, but instead I decide I have to know the truth.

"Do you want to sleep with me?"

Again, he starts mumbling and not really answering my question, so I decide to call his bluff. "Seriously. Do you want to sleep with me or not?"

"I do," he says sheepishly.

"Well, then why don't you go down to the store and buy some." He reaches to touch my shoulder and say something else, but I turn away. "I'm serious."

He cautiously backs away from me like a cowardly prince trying not to wake the dragon. Without another word, he puts on some jeans and a T-shirt and heads out of the room.

As l lie there alone in bed I start thinking about the whole dilemma. I feel like a bad *Afterschool Special.* Like we've both heard the slogan, "no glove, no love," too many times so we won't proceed without it. Usually in those specials, though, things work out and the girl always ends up happy, but that is not the case with me. In the TV version, Randy would come back, apologize for the mix-up, tell me he loves me for me, and then make love to me, but in this version I am alone and naked on a hotel bed and my arms are starting to go numb.

Great, I think, not only am I rejected by the man I like, but now my disease is acting up.

Luckily, 45 minutes later, Randy finally returns and so does the feeling in my fingers.

"So?" I ask, focusing on the real task at hand.

"They were closed."

"Then where'd you go?" I question.

"I looked around, but nothing was open. I couldn't find any anywhere."

Seriously? Are you kidding me?! Since when does Vegas not have condoms? But I have lost the strength to say more.

"I guess we should just go to sleep," I say, then turn my back to him and close my eyes. The room is silent but I can't seem to slip off into a quick slumber. My mind is racing and my body is aching.

I wonder if this is what blue balls feels like.

If so, this sucks, and I'd like to take this moment and apologize to all the boys I ever teased with my lips or otherwise. I'm truly sorry.

And now that I've gotten that out of the way, I'd like to take a little moment with God as well.

God, I know my body is fucked up and diseased, but besides my little lapse in judgment with Brad, I haven't had sex in months and now I'm horny and I need to make love... but apparently Vegas is not the place to go looking for romance. Apparently, when you start approaching 30, and you're living with a disabling disease and you might have cancer, what happens in Vegas is absolutely nothing.

Unless...

God is listening or I am dreaming. Because all of a sudden I am awoken from my slumber and I can feel Randy on top of me. The red of the clock blares out eight in the morning. The room is darkened by the thick shades. Our bodies are moving in synch. He has his boxers on, and we are dry humping.

Did I initiate this in my dreams? Did he initiate it? How are we in this position?

But I don't even care.

I go with it because it feels good and I think screw it, if we take this further he can just pull out. Not exactly the best method for pregnancy prevention but desperate times call for desperate measures. Besides, if I get knocked up that will be nine months without symptoms, which would mean so much more sleep for me, which would mean less bags under my eyes, which would mean Randy might want to do me more often, which would be okay since I'd already be pregnant, which would mean he'd have to marry me, which would mean I could stop dating, which would mean...

Yes, yes, oh...

No!

And just like that my fantasy is over. Because before he even gets close to entering me he is done.

Without a word he slips off into the bathroom to clean up the mess that is in his pants and I slip into sleep.

The drive home to LA is full of the silence that comes from a lack of sleep, a slight hangover, and a relationship fizzling.

I think this will be the end, but when we get close to Randy's place he announces his plan.

Plan B.

"What are we going to do about this morning?" he asks.

I look at him with a blank face. I don't know how to respond. Does he want me to tell him that it's okay? That it happens to a lot of guys?

"I think we should stop at the pharmacy," he says.

"Why do we need to stop?" I ask. Does he really think we can go buy condoms now and finally do it?

"You know, for the pill," he tells me.

"I told you I don't take it."

"Not *the* pill. The morning-after pill," he says, correcting his mistake.

"Oh, you mean Plan B?" I ask.

"We don't want to have a kid, do we?"

What the hell, you came in your pants. Not me.

"I guess not," I sigh, thinking this guy is seriously messed up. First there are rules on nakedness, then there is the lack of sex, then there's the no condom situation, and now he wants me to take emergency contraception on the off chance that he has some kind of super sperm that jumped from his boxers into my box.

I look over at Randy. His blonde hair and blue eyes would have made for perfect breeding, but there is no way I want to get pregnant with this man's child.

What if he does have sperm of steel?

"There's a Walgreens down the street from my place," I say.

And as I swallow the tiny white pills, I realize that some of the best-laid plans don't always include getting laid.

Chapter Nineteen

THOSE THREE WORDS
(Every Girl Wants to Hear)

There are three words that are far more life changing than "I love you," or "Let's make love" and today is the day I think I might hear them.

It is one week after Vegas. I'm cautiously sitting on the paper-covered exam table in my regular doctor's office as I wait for her to enter. My sweaty palms look pale and sickly under the fluorescent lights and the U Penn diploma on the wall does nothing to make me feel good about the *Us Weekly* in my hand. I'm waiting to receive the results of my thyroid ultrasound and I'm pretty convinced that the three words I'm about to hear today are:

You have cancer.

Which is why I'm still with Randy.

Several days after we returned from Sin City, he and I finally talked. I was seriously ready to walk away from our relationship, but Randy had an explanation as to why we weren't having sex. He told me that his good friend from law school, who was also about to take the bar, had accidentally gotten his girlfriend pregnant and after seeing how much his friend was struggling Randy didn't want to take that risk. He was about to become incredibly busy. He had to pass the bar. He couldn't complicate things. He didn't want to get me pregnant. Instead of taking that as a sign that we probably didn't have a future together, I re-interpreted his explanation as: One day he'd like to have kids with me but right now he needs to focus on his career so that when we do get married and have babies he'll be able to buy us a house and send our kids to private school and keep me in pretty jewels so we can't mess that up right now with an accidental pregnancy.

Looking at it that way, I'm completely content with the way things are between us.

If today is another day of bad news, I'm going to need Randy to come over. I'm going to need him to kiss me, touch me, hold me, hug me, sit with me. I don't need sex. I don't need a perfect relationship. I just need something that says, "You are still lovable."

I put the trashy magazine back in its proper holder on the wall and start to bounce my leg up and down out of nervousness. Finally, my doctor knocks on the door and enters with a smile on her face.

Her presence comforts me. The only good thing that's come out of all this medical mess is that my regular doctor is on my side. She actually remembers me when I visit and knows everything that's been going on without having to read my charts.

"So," she begins, "I hear they found some nodules on your thyroid and the MS specialist you see ordered an ultrasound."

"Yes, and they were supposed to send the results here."

"Unfortunately, we never got any reports or results."

What? How can that be? You were supposed to tell me that I have cancer. Or I don't. But you were supposed to tell me something.

"Now what?" I ask, thinking this is never going to end. I'm going to have to come back here and worry about the results all over again. Maybe I should've sworn off doctors forever, not just for Lent.

"Well, you'll have to call over to UCLA and get them to send you your report and then you can send it to me here and we can figure out the next step."

"The next step?" Awesome. She thinks it's cancer too.

"Don't worry," she starts, sensing my fear. "Most of the time these nodules are benign, but if they're over one centimeter in diameter then we usually like to biopsy them, just in case. And how's everything else?"

I tell her things are as good as they can be and give her the latest update on my recent MRIs and appointments, I tell her about the evoked potentials and the fact that the specialist still thinks I have MS, but is waiting for that last bit of clinical proof.

"I can't even imagine what you're going through. Are you sleeping okay?"

"Umm, well…," I start, almost wanting to tell her everything as if she's my best friend. I wonder what she'd say if I was honest and told her, well, yes actually, I sleep great. In fact I sleep all the time, mostly during the day. But that's probably because I don't sleep much at night since the numbness and pain in my arms usually wakes me up. Also I have this new addiction to the internet and I now have this fear of waking immobile so I stay up late researching my symptoms. Oh, and then there's this guy I like, who I probably shouldn't, but I do anyway because I don't want to face this alone so I keep him around even though he doesn't want to sleep with me and I haven't had sex in too many months to count and I'm starting to feel like I may never do it again, but yeah, besides all that I'm sleeping just great.

"I know you don't like to take drugs, but I can prescribe some Ambien if you want."

I pause for a second and think about accepting her offer, the thought of a good night's sleep sounds amazing, but I can't do it. I really do hate drugs and I have a huge aversion to their side effects, especially the ones that tell me I may start eating in my sleep or saying crazy things, which is almost as bad as the other drugs the neurologist offered me that warned of rapid weight gain.

"No, that's okay," I say with the broad smile and chipper voice I've gotten used to presenting to everyone around me. I tell her how I've been doing a lot of yoga lately and it seems to help. Then I add that I've been eating really well too. Mainly organic. I sit up straighter on the table and hope she buys my story and my facade of confidence.

"Good, I'm glad."

"So, I guess we'll do this again soon?" I ask, as if I'm so excited about coming back to hear whether or not I've got cancer.

"Yeah. Call UCLA, get the report, and then I'll call you once you send it to me and we'll figure this out. I'm sure it's nothing. Hang in there," she says as she smiles and leaves.

I take a look again at her diploma on the wall and remember my own childhood dream of becoming a doctor. I wonder if I'd majored in biology instead of creative writing if things would be different. If instead of writing about all my medical experiences I'd be looking for my own cure.

For a second I think about calling my bosses and telling them I'm done with Hollywood, I'm over being a writer and I'm going back to school to become a doctor. Of course, I don't actually do this but I do pick up my phone and call the UCLA ultrasound center as I head out of the doctor's office.

Immediately I am put on hold.

Elevator music plays in my ear as I begin the drive back home down the Pacific Coast. The annoying sounds add to my frustrations. I look out the window at the beach below to try to calm me, but after five minutes I've had enough.

I open my mouth and scream into the empty air of the car. *What the fuck?! Is this crap ever going to end? Ahhhhhhh hhhhhhhhhhhhhhhhhhhhhhhhhhhhhhhhh...*

Suddenly, the light ahead of me turns red, I am jolted out of my thoughts, and I slam on the brakes. My car skids to a screeching halt and my gaze travels from the sea below to the sign above. I am at the corner of Ocean and Wilshire. I take another look at the beach to the right and steal a glance at the line of cars to the left. It suddenly becomes clear what I am to do today. I have two choices: I can live with the thoughts that come with uncertainty, or I can find an answer.

The UCLA center that has put me on hold lies 16 blocks to the east. My apartment is a ten-minute drive south. I could go home, call my parents, and cry, then sit around all day wondering why. Or I could figure this out on my own.

As the light turns green I make my decision. I hang up the phone, put my car in gear, grip the wheel, and make a hard left. I speed out of there like Mario Andretti, buzz past a Mercedes, and nearly blow through a red.

Sixteen blocks later I find myself parked around the corner from the beige brick building where I once sat amidst a group of expectant moms all waiting to see pictures of their in-utero babies.

I hop out of my car, scour my purse for dimes and quarters, and feed the meter until the blinking display stops flashing and lets me know I have exactly one hour and eight minutes to enter the premises, secure the data, and exit unscathed.

As I approach the front door, I remove the Ray-Ban aviators from my eyes and steel myself to begin Operation Cancer Discovery. I head straight to the ultrasound room of the medical center and saddle up to the front desk like I mean business.

"Can I help you?" the overweight woman behind the desk asks me.

"Yes. Yes you can," I respond with some newfound authority that doesn't really sound like me whatsoever.

"Okay, do you have an appointment?"

"No, no," I begin as I take a look at all the knocked up women around me, the same kind of women who ostracized me the last time I visited this center. "I was here two weeks ago. They were supposed to send my results to my doctor, but they didn't, so I'd like a copy."

"We don't have that here," she answers quickly, as if to say "everyone knows that."

I ask her where I can get them.

She pauses for a second before answering then holds up her hand to tell me to wait a minute as she pours a handful of M&Ms into her palm from the little candy dispenser on her desk.

With a mouth full of fat and high fructose corn syrup she tells me that the records department holds all records.

I ask her where that is as I watch her continue to shove the chocolate candies into her mouth.

"Go back down the hall you came in, turn right, follow that hallway 'til it ends, then make another right and you'll be there."

I turn to leave and start to walk away when I catch the eye of one of the expectant mothers. I take a moment and pause and think about being nice and asking her when she's due, but instead I look straight at her husband and flash him a great big smile. She glares at me, but I just nod, *Yeah, I'm looking at your man.* Then I take off down the hall and head for the records department.

When I enter the stark white room with its tall black desk, my heart begins to beat faster. I am literally moments away from discovering whether or not I have cancer and the cocky confident facade I had minutes earlier has completely disappeared. I contemplate walking out the door, calling the center, waiting on hold for hours, having the reports sent here or there, letting the doctors track me down, allowing things to happen in a nice bureaucratic fashion, the way the system wants you to do it, but I've already decided today's the day I go against the grain and take matters into my own hands. Operation Cancer Discovery, aka OCD, will continue on as planned.

I wait a few minutes for the woman to return to the front desk and I begin, "Hi, I'm here, for, uh, the, uh, thing, that I, uh." Oh God, now I know why they ask you to follow the rules and not try to do this by yourself. I can't even talk like a normal human being. I'm stuttering like a teenage girl called upon in class by the hot teacher. "I, uh, have results, that, uh, I need," I finally manage to spit out.

"Ultrasound, MRI, CAT Scan, or Xray?"

"Ultrasound," I mutter.

"Great. I need you to fill out this form so that we can release a copy to you. You want the images on a CD, right?"

I hadn't even thought about it but, "Yes. That's fine," I tell the woman as I fill in my name, address, and social security number and hand her back the form.

She tells me it will cost 15 dollars and should only take ten minutes. I hand her the money and she exits through a "Staff Only" door to retrieve my results.

I take a seat in a white plastic chair against the bare wall in the waiting area. The room is empty except for me. I keep one eye on the door where the woman disappeared and the other on my watch. A minute goes by, then another, and I start to feel the open emptiness of the room. For the first time I am absolutely, completely alone. Sure, I've gone to other appointments by myself, but there has always been at least two other people in the waiting room with me, and there's usually a receptionist and people coming and going, but this room is dead quiet.

At first I think nothing of it and enjoy the stillness, but then it hits me. My OCD mission might be one of the dumbest things I've decided to do in my entire life. I'm about to find out if I have cancer and if I actually do no one's going to be here to help me process the bad news. I will have no one to turn to. No doctor will follow the diagnosis with a sympathetic "I'm sorry," or an explanation or a plan to defeat it, my parents won't be able to hold me, and there will be no Randy or any other man by my side to tell me it will be okay. I am literally going to have to deal with it all on my own.

I contemplate running out the door and never looking back. No one would even notice and if it's cancer the doctors will eventually track me down and if it's not then it's no big deal anyway. I look towards the front door and start to inch off my seat, but something stops me. A strange weight seems to be holding me back, it's a feeling in my gut that seems to be telling me that I can't go this far and not finish my mission. I have to face the truth and I have to do it alone. If I can't do this right here, right now, then I'm never going to be able to live with any of this medical stuff no matter how healthy or sick or single or betrothed I eventually become.

I glance down at my watch. T minus five minutes until the woman returns with my results. My leg begins to nervously bounce up and down. My palms begin to sweat. I take a few deep breaths, but my heart is pounding and my lungs feel tight.

Finally, the woman returns.

"Here's your ultrasound," she says as she hands me a CD.

I reach out and grab the paper sleeve and quickly pull out the disc. But the only things on the CD are my name and birth date printed neatly across the front. I flip it over and look inside the sleeve, but there's nothing else.

"Uh, are the results printed somewhere that I can't see?" I ask.

"Oh, no," she smiles. "This is just your ultrasound itself. If you want the radiologist's report you're going to have to go across the street to the hospital. On the second floor is the written records department and they'll have a copy there."

I exit the room and head down the hallway. I am completely confused, should I go across the street and finish this mission or should I take this as a sign and let the doctors handle it? I finally reach the door that leads to the outside of the building and look across to the hospital. The sun beats down on me and I think about what to do next. Then I make my decision.

I have to get the results. I shove the CD in my purse, put on my sunglasses, and quickly cross the street before I have time to change my mind.

I race past closed doors and families looking for loved ones. The smell of Band-Aids and latex and cheap cleaning solvent fills the air. My Converse sneakers squeak on the cold sterile floor. The place is a labyrinth of disease and unanswered questions, but I continue charging forward. As I round the corner, I hear the elevator doors ding open. I rush to them but am forced to pause as an elderly man with tubes and wires protruding from his body is wheeled out in front of me. The male nurse gives me a smile as he pushes the hospital bed out of the elevator and down the hall away from me. I hop in the massive cabin and hit the button for the second floor.

The elevator slowly moves up and I can feel my stomach drop like it used to do when I was a kid and my sister and I would jump in the elevator before it stopped and we'd feel a moment of weightlessness. When the elevator reaches the second floor, I exit and turn to the right. Finally, I round the corner and see it, like a white light at the end of a tunnel, the room I have been looking for.

There, behind the sliding glass window where an administrator sits is my destiny. I quickly walk to the written records department and approach the woman behind the glass.

"I need to get the report on an ultrasound," I tell her.

"Sure, I just need your name, birth date, social, address, and date of service."

I supply her with all of this information and she quickly types it into her computer.

"I found it," she says and I expect her to say that she needs to go to some dark back room and retrieve the records, and it will take at least an hour and if I'd like to go grab some lunch or check out the gift shop she'll have it ready when I return, but then I hear her printer whir to life and in less than 30 seconds flat she hands me the report.

"That's it?"

"That's it," she says.

I slowly grab the paper and my hand immediately begins to shake.

I turn and walk away so that the woman does not have to see my sense of unease. I start to read as I walk back to the elevator.

Bilateral thyroid cysts are identified. At least two such cysts are present on the right measuring up to 8mm, and two such cysts are present on the left, measuring up to 11mm.

I nearly drop the paper on the floor. There are four cysts? I only thought there was one. This cannot be good. My gait slows as I let the news sink in. How can this be true? But then I pause and remember that my doctor said the cysts would only have to be biopsied if they were over one centimeter, anything smaller than that was not a concern. Then I get mad at the fact that I haven't taken math since high school. How many millimeters are in a centimeter? Ten? A hundred? Does it even go that way? I can't remember. I don't know. I start to panic.

I have cancer. I have cancer.

My eyes begin to well and my feet start to drag. This is it. This is the end. This is how it happens. Me, alone, in a dark hospital hallway slumped on the floor in tears. Dim yellow lights above me. An eerie silence.

Oh God. Oh God.

I hold the paper up overhead closer to the light. Maybe there's a hidden message. Something new. Something that's better.

This cannot be happening. Not here. Not right now. Why didn't I wait and let the doctor give me this news? Why didn't I ask someone to go with me? Why did I feel like I had something to prove?

I'm about to totally lose it when I notice more writing at the bottom of the paper.

Impression: Bilateral sub and peri-centimeter thyroid cysts as described, benign appearing.

It takes me a minute to process, but I know what those words mean. I'm free.

I don't have cancer.

The point is proven. The test is passed. I am strong and I've just seen the two best words in my life.

Benign. Appearing.

I smile then exit the hospital and head to my car. I start the engine, turn up the radio, and open the windows.

I let the wind blow through my hair as I drive back down Wilshire and head toward the beach. The salty air nips at the corner of my results as they peek out of my purse. My passenger seat sits empty, and I rejoice, because today I am happy, healthy, and alive.

When I talk to Randy later that evening, I make no mention of the cancer scare. He goes off to study for the bar and our relationship begins to fade. Six weeks later we make one last attempt at dinner, but when he cancels to help his aunt with her divorce, I take it as a sign that Randy's only real strength lies in annulling relationships, not creating them.

Part 2

Chapter Twenty

PAPER COVERS ROCK

I definitely should have gone to med school because last night I made a new medical discovery: Sex with a doctor can have serious side effects.

How do I know this? The scientific method of course.

That and the fact that the guy I banged in the wee hours of the morning was a doctor and now I'm having second thoughts.

Yes, in its most classical form, I had a one-night stand. No, I don't do that sort of thing all the time. And, yes, I've got some serious issues. But I can explain, or at least I can try.

Yesterday, October 16, 2008, marked the one-year anniversary of my diagnosis. As an important milestone in my life, I'd decided that, instead of sulking at home feeling sorry for myself, it was time to make a change. This date would no longer be forever dark as the day I received bad news, I was now calling it my Lesion-Stable Anniversary. The five original lesions they had found on my brain still remained, but, according to a more recent MRI, no new ones had appeared over the last 365 days—and that was a very good thing. Add that to the fact that I didn't have cancer and I had had the courage to end things with Randy, and my perspective on life with the disease was beginning to change. Negative test results and no new symptoms were now a positive sign that if I did truly have MS then it wasn't as bad as it could be and that was cause for celebration. In order to acknowledge my new perspective and my anniversary with MS, I decided to invite a few friends out for drinks.

When we arrived at the bar it was fairly quiet. There wasn't much going on except loud music and a couple of older long-haired surfer dudes drinking in the back.

My friends and I grabbed a table in the corner and chatted and enjoyed our drinks. We cheered to good health, and laughed about our days. A night out with friends was exactly what I needed.

Of course, one hour and one beer later that all changed when a group of three very attractive guys entered the bar. I tried to avoid eye contact because this was supposed to be a girls' night, but ten minutes later they were at our table.

"What are you ladies doing out on a Thursday?" one of the cute guys asked.

My friend Jen looked at me to take the lead.

"Oh, you know, it's been a rough week at work," I said. While I had accepted the fact that MS was a part of my life, I still didn't feel the need to broadcast it to the world, or every good-looking guy I met.

"What do you girls do?" another asked.

My friends said, "PR," "medical sales," and I made up some story about what I did for a living, and quickly turned the tables. "And you guys?"

"We're doctors. Residents actually. It's the first night we've had off in weeks," said the last guy with beautiful green eyes.

I looked at him and thought how convenient or ironic it was that on my one-year Lesion-Stable Anniversary I would meet a doctor. For a second I felt like I could be the subject of some Alanis Morissette song and at any moment the guys would tell me they were MS specialists.

"What kind of doctors are you?" Colleen asked.

"We work in the ER," he said.

I looked at the green-eyed stud and made a mental note that if I ever had a medical emergency I would go to their hospital.

"Do you want another drink?" he asked me. I looked down and saw that my glass was empty and said sure.

The doctor and I wandered to the bar and grabbed two more beers. We quickly settled in to a light conversation. I gazed at his brilliant eyes and noted his high level of education. I asked him about the craziest things he'd seen in the emergency room. He went on about car crashes and burns, bullet wounds and heart attacks. I mentioned nothing of my own medical stories. Soon, our friends joined us and we all clinked glasses in recognition of meeting new people and before we knew it the lights came on and the bartenders announced the place was closing.

"Do you guys want to go back to my place for a night-cap?" I asked my friends and the doctors. They all declined saying they had to work. But me? I was free to keep going. This was a perk of working from home. I could go out on a weeknight and not have to worry about waking early the next day to report to an office, and I didn't want the party to end.

"Are you sure?" I tried once more.

Everyone shook their heads, but then...

"Um, you know what, I'd like another drink," the doctor I'd been chatting with earlier said.

I was surprised. We had had a nice conversation, but I didn't think he'd want to go home with me. Or at least not alone. This wasn't a "hang out and make out" kind of situation. However, since it was a night to celebrate, I figured, *Why the hell not?* and the doctor and I took a cab back to my place.

In my mind I pictured the rendezvous at my apartment to be very PG. We'd have a couple drinks and listen to some music. Perhaps we'd share a kiss or two and then I'd get tipsy, spill my guts about the MS, and he'd give me a hug, tell me it'd be okay and that would be that. We'd probably become friends for a few years afterwards and he'd keep me abreast of any new research or drugs I could take, I'd feed him my ideas for other cures and he'd give them due diligence, and when he met the woman of his dreams I'd be cast aside and grateful he had come into my life. Our relationship would be very easy. And that's why I only had one intention for that evening and that was to keep the party going.

But the doctor had other intentions.

When we got back to my place, I let him enter first then closed the door behind us. As I turned to offer him a drink, he abruptly pulled me in for a kiss.

I was completely caught off guard and stood stunned for a second.

"I'm sorry," he said.

"Um, no, it was just… that was unexpected…"

"What about this?"

He kissed me again and I started to hesitate, but this time when his soft lips gently pressed into mine, I didn't pull away.

"Okay, that was okay," I said as we stopped.

"And this?"

He pulled me closer and kissed me harder, and suddenly any innocent ideas I'd had about the evening went out the window. I don't know if it was some sort of doctor/fireman rescue me fantasy being played out but I went with it.

I wrapped my arms around him then melted into his chest. It was magical or, to be more concise, it lit the fire in my loins. Shit. I was horny. But why? This guy was supposed to be the life of the party, not another notch on the belt. And then I realized, not only had it been a year since my diagnosis, it had also been quite a while since I'd been laid. Then I thought, this had to be more than an ironic coincidence. It had to mean something. So, I kissed him again to make sure.

For years my family has joked that I've kissed a lot of frogs looking for my prince. Always kissing frogs hoping some spell will be lifted, but last night I thought perhaps it would be the reverse, and if I let the boy kiss me maybe the spell of MS would be gone, or at least the spell of abstinence.

"Come here," he said, pulling me closer.

The doctor's hands continued to wander my body. Gently, we plucked away each other's clothing and before I knew it we were naked in bed.

I paused for a moment. Did I really want to break the spell with a one-night stand? The doctor and I knew very little about each other and the only thing we had in common was that he practiced medicine and I was in need of medicine. Then I thought maybe this was exactly the right way to do it. For once since the diagnosis, I could get laid. And this prescription of fornication would come without side effects. It would be no-strings-attached sex. He would just be a means to an end. The end of my dry spell. I let out a sigh of relief as he made his way on top of me. If there were ever an appropriate time to pull off a one-night stand it would be with Dr. Stranger.

I let the man work his magic. In, out; harder, faster. Our bodies crashed together and I felt safe, that no matter what happened the MD could take care of it, because that's what he did for a living.

This morning? Well, that's a different story.

After a night of carnal fun, Dr. One Nighter and I wake up in my bed to discover there is a big problem with our situation. Without going into exact details, let's just say the chances of a twice-used fully loaded condom springing a leak are pretty high, and now the doctor has questions.

"When was the first day of your last period?"

I think for a moment then respond, "last Tuesday."

"Are you pretty regular?"

"Yes. Twenty-eight days usually," I say, then think how clinical the whole situation feels and how odd it is that I barely know this guy and now he knows the ins and outs of my lady cycle.

"Well, you're not at your most fertile, but we should get emergency contraception just in case," the doctor says.

"Okay," I reply, realizing that I am once again in a situation where I have to buy the morning-after pill, only this time I had actually had sex.

I can't believe this is happening for the second time in a span of six months and think how much easier life would be if I could be on normal birth control. Then, when I had drunken one-night stands, or got dry humped in Vegas, I wouldn't have to admit my mistakes and wrong choices in men to the pharmacist doling out the levonorgestrel.

"I'll go with you to Walgreens," the doctor says, "then you can drop me off at my place afterwards."

"Ummm, that would be a great plan," I say, "if I hadn't left my car at the bar last night."

Clearly, we hadn't thought through our sexcapade, because had we made better arrangements he would've woken this morning, kissed me on the forehead, whispered "last night was fun," then quietly slipped out my door. I would've been cured of my celibacy and there would've been no repercussions to our actions.

Instead, we now have to spend the next hour together in awkwardness.

Once we both re-dress ourselves, we decide it makes the most sense to walk to his place near the beach, get his hybrid, go to the pharmacy, and pick up my Jeep afterwards.

After a 15-minute stroll in near silence, we finally make it to his apartment, get his car, and drive to the store. His Prius purrs to a stop in the parking lot. Slowly he looks at me with his bright green eyes and I am reminded why I'd let him enter me. He is hot, and the sex was good. Maybe this isn't so bad.

But then he says, "We both don't have to go in, do we?"

"Umm," I hesitate, "I guess not." *But it'd be nice.*

When he sees my look of concern, I think he is going to volunteer to go with me, however, this is what I get instead: "How 'bout we rock, paper, scissors for it?"

"Seriously?" I ask.

"Yeah, why not?"

Because we did this together. Because you're an ass if you don't. Because... I could go on, but why should you argue with a guy you know you're never going to see again?

"Fine," I state, figuring that at least I'd have a 50 percent chance of winning.

"On the count of three, we go."

One. Two. Three.

We both display our hands. I go rock. He goes paper. Fuck. Paper covers rock.

I walk the 50 feet to the store and ignore the homeless man asking for cash as I approach the door. My heart starts to beat a nervous patter as soon as I enter. Suddenly, the Catholic girl in me feels guilty. Not because I slept with a total stranger I met at a bar the night before, not because I couldn't remember his name—Andrew, Alex, Axl?—and not because I was about to take some high-dose hormones to make sure I didn't get knocked up. I had committed the ultimate sin. I'd had premarital sex and in my mind that was worse. Even though I had lost my virginity years ago and stopped going to church midway through high school, whenever I had to admit to authorities or adults that I was doing it without lifelong commitment I resorted to being a 13-year-old girl waiting for marriage. I always felt like I had done the worst thing possible. To cover my indiscretion, I meander the aisles, pretending to be looking for new shampoo or a tube of lipstick. And because I'm not wearing any jewelry, I wander down the toy aisle and contemplate buying one of the princess dress-up rings and placing it on my ring finger so that people will think I am married, or at the very least engaged. But I'm pretty sure plastic does not pass for diamond. So instead I am stuck confessing to the world that I was a sinner.

As I wonder how many Our Fathers and Hail Marys it would take to absolve me of this sin, the pharmacy area comes into view.

I check to see if there is anyone I know lurking around the enemas in the corner, or the tampons in the next aisle. I look left, then right, then see the coast is clear. I make a mad dash to the counter.

"Can I help you?" the pharmacist asks.

"Do you have Plan B?" I try to say with confidence, but I am certain my voice sounds like a pre-pubescent boy's.

She nods, then quickly goes to the shelves of drugs and pulls out the little blue and white box.

That was easy, I think. *This woman is good. No judgment. Nothing. Maybe I won't have to go to hell after all.*

"I'll need to see your ID," she says.

What? I want to yell: *I'm not trying to get drunk, that's what got me here in the first place.* But then I remember that you have to be 18 to buy the pill and suddenly I am flattered that she doesn't think I am of age. Of course, it also crosses my mind that if this were true, she probably thinks I acted in one of those "barely legal" films last night, where it was all boobs, bad dialogue, and hard pounding.

"Your total's $52.78," the pharmacist says.

I swipe my debit card, okay the amount, then realize that in some convoluted way I've just paid for sex. Happy one-year anniversary to me.

The pharmacist hands me a small white bag and I turn to leave.

"How'd it go?" the doctor asks when I return to the car.

"Fine. I got carded."

"Oh, I probably should've written you a prescription," he says nonchalantly.

"That might've been a good idea," I answer. "Since I could've used my insurance then, but that's fine. What's 50 bucks?"

"Sorry," he says. "Maybe next—" But he cuts himself off because the truth is we both know exactly what this was and there will not be a next time.

I turn and look out the window as he quietly starts the car. I sit in my seat and silently watch the buildings roll by.

When we finally get to my car back at the bar, we say our good-byes and awkwardly hug. Then he points to the bag in my hand and says, "Make sure you take those on time."

Once I get home, I flip on the TV and settle onto my couch with a nice glass of water. I open the box of two pills and swallow the first one with a big gulp. As it goes down my throat, I imagine it to be a panacea for all my ills, then I set the alarm on my phone to go off in 12 hours so I don't miss the second one. After all it was the doctor's orders and if doctors don't know it all, then who does?

Chapter Twenty-One

SPINAL TAP

The next time a man tells me it's not going to hurt because he's going to go slow and make sure I'm ready, I'm running in the opposite direction.

I should've learned this lesson in college when my boyfriend at the time suggested we try anal sex. We were young and naive and experimenting and he told me it would be fine. Two seconds later I was screaming "STOP!"

There are some things that are not meant to be entered. One of which is my behind, the other of which is my spinal column.

Yes, spinal column. Oh come on, you didn't really think I was going to write a whole chapter on entering through the back door did you? That's gross.

Instead I'd like to tell you the tale of my lumbar puncture, otherwise known as a spinal tap.

It's November 2008, more than a year since this medical journey began. I've been shocked and scanned and sat in front of a screen of blinking, checkered-like blocks and yet, while the specialist still believes I have the disease, she can't give me the one hundred percent diagnosis until she gets one last piece of clinical evidence. And that's where the spinal tap comes in.

In 80 percent of MS patients the cerebral spinal fluid shows something called oligoclonal bands (o-bands) that have a higher amount of certain proteins that indicate the breakdown of the myelin sheath that covers nerves and is indicative of the body attacking itself.

Because I'm tired of living in a state of limbo where I don't quite know where I stand when it comes to this lovely disease of mine, at my regular appointment I finally agree to do the test.

"Great," the specialist says, then turns to the resident who's been allowed to observe my exam, "Do you want to do it?"

The resident, who's probably in his early thirties and looks like a bona fide dork, takes one look at me and my young supple spine and the smile on his face indicates that it's clear he's just won the Mega Millions jackpot. For a moment I feel like I'm in an episode of some bad medical drama and I am no longer a person, but a specimen ready to be tested so that the student can brag to his colleagues about the rare procedure he got to perform.

"You're not going to do it today are you?" I ask, afraid the resident is going to get trigger happy with a needle right then and there in the office.

"No," my doctor explains, "you and Dr. Chan can set up a time for next week. He'll tell you everything you need to know for before and after the test."

"Okay," I say with hesitation.

"Don't worry," she says, "it's not as scary as you think. I promise."

She gives me a smile, shakes my hand, and exits the room. Dr. Chan and I stare at each other for a moment until he breaks the silence.

"Let's go see the receptionist in scheduling so we can find a time next week that works."

I follow Dr. Chan out of the sterile grey and white exam room and down the hall to scheduling. When we arrive at the desk there are several patients in front of us. As we wait for our turn he begins to give me the lowdown on my spinal tap.

He makes it sound super simple. All I have to do is show up, he'll numb the area, stick the needle in, draw some fluid, and several minutes later I'll be done.

"The only thing we ask is that you lie flat on your back for at least eight hours after the procedure, so that the puncture can heal properly."

"You can't just put a Band-Aid on it?" I ask, thinking it's one small needle going in between my vertebrae, why would I need to lie down?

"We will put a Band-Aid on it. But the place where the needle enters into the sac around your spinal column needs to close up. Cerebral spinal fluid doesn't clot like blood and we've found that if patients lie flat on their back it heals quicker."

"Oh," I mumble, realizing that this may be a bigger deal than I thought. "Then I guess I'll buy a bunch of magazines and plan an afternoon on my couch catching up on celebrity gossip and watching trashy TV," I say in an attempt to lighten the mood.

However, the doctor apparently could not care less about the *Real Housewives,* and when I look up at him I realize it's our turn and he's already looking at next week's schedule.

"So, how about Tuesday at one-thirty?" he asks.

"Ummm, well, I guess that will work. I mean I don't have anything scheduled. But will I need someone to drive me?"

"Do you have a partner?" I shake my head no. "How about a friend?"

"All of my friends work."

"Hmmmm…" The wheels in Dr. Chan's head start to spin and so do mine.

"Do I have to do it next week?" I ask. "I mean I can probably get my parents to fly out here if I give them a little bit more notice."

Dr. Chan looks at me, then answers. "That'd be silly. That's a lot to spend on a flight for a little test."

"I know, but I don't think they'd care."

Dr. Chan shakes his head again. "Nah. How about we push it to next Friday and maybe you can get a friend to take off work at lunch time?"

"Ummmm," I start to say something like, *No, I'd rather wait until I can get a proper ride.* But have I told you how bad I am with salesmen and saying no? Dr. Chan's ready to sell me a needle in my spine and I'm buying it like it's the next SlimFast.

"Okay. Next Friday is fine," I say, hoping that I can convince someone to take off work and help me out.

"And if you can't find someone to drive you, we can make it work."

"Can I stay overnight upstairs?" I ask, knowing that just floors above me is the UCLA hospital and I would feel better if I had 'round-the-clock care.

"No, that's not necessary. When I'm done performing the puncture we can put you in one of our extra exam rooms and then after an hour or two lying there you should be ready to go. How far do you live from here?"

"Twenty minutes. Without traffic," I say matter of fact, trying to ignore his suggestion that lying in a dark room by myself is going to be perfect.

"You should be fine. The car ride shouldn't affect the healing process."

"I don't know," I say, feeling a pit start to rise in my stomach. "I think I'd rather wait and have my parents fly out here."

"I swear it'll go by so quickly, it'll be like nothing happened."

And before I can gather the strength to tell him no, I'd like to wait, the receptionist hands me a piece of paper with my appointment date and time on it.

"I'll see you next week," Dr. Chan says.

I nod okay, then in a haze start to walk away. I turn back for a second to see if I can change my mind but Dr. Chan gives me a smile and a little wave good-bye and I am surprised to see that there on his ring finger is a nice gold band.

How can this man think it'd be a great idea for me to lie alone in an exam room dripping fluids from my back? What if it was his wife? Would he just leave her? And what if one day he has a daughter? Would he leave her? Who knows, but I can guarantee this resident was raised by a tiger mom.

When I return home that afternoon I call my own mom. I tell her that I have finally agreed to do the spinal tap.

"Are you sure you want to do it?" she asks.

"Yes," I reply, "I'm tired of waiting. If the test comes back positive then I'll know for sure I have MS."

"What if it comes back negative?"

I pause for a second. For the last year of my life I've been struggling to come to grips with the reality that I have MS, but...

"It never occurred to you that you might *not* have it, did it?" she asks.

"No. Because I know there's something wrong with me," I snap at her. It isn't that I want to have the disease, it's that I've spent over 12 months creating a new reality for my world. A reality where I know that at any moment my body could fail me and my limbs could be rendered useless.

Which is why I am doing yoga five times a week and standing on my head, taking lifts to double-black-diamond ski slopes and passing signs that warn experts only, hopping behind a boat and wakeboarding for the first time in eight years. It is also why I can't sleep at night and take baclofen to relax my muscles, why I will never try Bikram and have to leave yoga if the room gets too hot. It is why I struggle with relationships in a way that most girls will never have to. It is my reality. But a reality without MS? That I don't know. Even if I try to erase all I've been through and chalk it up to a doctor's mistake, I will always see the world in a different way. It is like the first time my mom told me what "making love" was in the fourth grade and every time after that when I saw adults who were married or had children all I could think about was the fact that that man probably stuck his penis in that woman's vagina the night before.

"You're really going to let them stick a needle in your spine?" my mom asks, interrupting my train of thought.

I explain to her that it doesn't seem so bad. When Dr. Comer wanted to do it a year ago she told me that it was just like getting an epidural, only instead of sticking the needle past the vertebrae and injecting the medicine outside the spinal column, they stick it in a little further and take out some fluid. "How bad can it be?"

"I don't know. I never had an epidural with you or your sister."

"Well, plenty of women do it and the resident said I'd be fine," I say quickly, clearly trying to convince myself more than my mom that this is not a big deal at all.

"How are you going to get home?"

"I'll drive."

"Really? When is your appointment again?"

"Next Friday at one."

She pauses and I can hear a door open.

"Okay, your dad just walked in—can I call you in a little bit?"

"Sure," I say, a bit peeved that she has to get off the phone so quickly.

But ten minutes later my mom calls me back to say that she and my dad have booked a flight and they will be in LA on Thursday to take me to my appointment on Friday.

"Thank you," I say, then thank God for my family as I hang up the phone with "I love you."

By the time the following Friday comes around I feel confident that the spinal tap will go off without a hitch. My parents and I are just about out the door when...

"You did remember to wear your pretty underwear, right?" my dad asks, remembering the story I'd told him of the cute technician who'd run my evoked potential tests.

"Yes, dad, they're fine," I say, knowing full well that the guy performing the procedure is neither hot nor single. Hence, the reason why I am wearing cotton short-like briefs that are more boyish and less sexy.

The drive from the Marina to Westwood is fairly quiet except for the directions I give from the back seat of the minivan my parents have rented—yes, my dad thinks it's cool to drive a minivan in LA because it's so unexpected and frankly, he likes to pull up to nice restaurants and ask them to keep it up front.

By the time we get to the bottom floor of Building 300 and I sign in at the front desk my heart is racing. Without saying a word my mom grabs my hand and we sit in the black chairs of the waiting room. I try to read *Time* or *Newsweek* and pretend I am interested, but clearly I have other things on my mind, like needles and spinal fluid and...

"Miss Martin, you ready?"

Dr. Chan appears at the door in all his over-achiever glory.

I nod, then stand up to follow him. As I kiss my parents good-bye, Dr. Chan turns and tells them, "I'll come and get you when we're done and you can sit with her while she recovers."

Before I know it I am lying on my side on a cold exam table, my pants are unbuttoned, my top is off and a paper gown is draped over my front. Dr. Chan grabs a sterile gauze and begins lubing up my back with iodine.

When he's covered every bit of my skin, he asks me to pull my knees in to my chest so that he can get a good look at my vertebrae. He starts palpating the bones with his latex covered fingers, pausing as he clearly counts up from my coccyx to find the perfect point of entry.

"You've got good muscle tone and are pretty fit. This will make it a lot easier," he says.

"What?"

"Sometimes with larger patients it's hard to find the spine and the space between the vertebrae."

"Oh," I say, then wonder if that's supposed to be some sort of compliment on my physique. Then I think about his wife and wonder if the first time they got naked together and he rode her from behind he started screaming things like, "Oh, baby, your body is so hot. Do you know how easy it would be to puncture your spine? Your vertebrae are so easy to find."

I feel Dr. Chan stop somewhere towards my lower spine then he says, "The first needle is going to numb the area. In a couple seconds you're going to feel a little pinch."

After what feels like a baby crab grabbing my back, he lets me lie on the table for a few minutes as the novocain or whatever other drug he used begins to take effect.

"Can you feel this?" he asks.

I can tell he's close to me and probably touching my back but I hardly feel a thing.

"Are you ready then?"

"I guess so," I respond, then close my eyes and take a deep cleansing breath.

"I need you to stay as still as possible," he says. "One more second and you'll feel some pressure. You're doing good."

Suddenly I feel this pressing feeling in my back as if someone is violating my spine. I want to scream but instead I take a few more breaths and wait in stillness until Dr. Chan gives me the okay to move.

When it's over, he places a tiny Band-Aid over the wound then tells me to roll over and lie flat.

"You're all done. See, it wasn't so bad was it?"

"Can you go get my parents?"

"Of course," he says gently and pats my shoulder, showing his first ounce of compassion since I'd met him.

A minute later, my parents arrive and sit in the two waiting chairs against the opposite wall.

"How was it?" my dad asks.

"Fine. I didn't really feel it. Though he did tell me I had a skinny spine, so I guess that was nice."

I look to my mom to see her reaction, but she's frozen silent. In a situation like this she'd normally ask me if the doctor was single or my age or something else embarrassing, but all she can do is keep staring at my torso and buttocks area.

"What are you looking at? Is my underwear hanging out or something?"

"No. It's..."

Then I look down and see that the paper covering the table is covered in a dark reddish brown fluid. "Oh my God. That's iodine, not blood."

"Oh good," she says, finally relaxing.

"Wait, were you going to sit there and look at it and not say anything?"

"I didn't want to freak you out. But you look good."

Just then Dr. Chan knocks on the door and enters.

"How did she do?" my dad asks.

"She did great. Just make sure when she gets home that she stays lying on her back for at least eight hours and if she starts to get a headache we recommend caffeine, a Coke or a soda usually does the trick."

"That's it?" my mom asks, resuming her role as caretaker as if I were her sick kid again, struggling to breathe with pneumonia.

"She should be fine. But there is one complication you need to know about. If she starts to experience massive headaches that are only relieved when she's lying down it means the puncture hasn't healed properly and you'll need to take her to the emergency room for a blood patch."

"Seriously?" I ask.

"Don't worry, it rarely ever happens. I promise," Dr. Chan says. "Just make sure you stay on your back for at least the rest of the afternoon."

Once we return to my apartment, my mom makes up the couch into a comfy little bed and I lie down on my back as she rubs my head. After an hour or so I drift off to sleep with the thought that at least the worst is over. I no longer have to see Dr. Chan, and my spine and anything else near my behind is again off limits.

Around six that evening, I awake to the orange sky reflecting off the marina water outside my window.

"How are you feeling?" my mom asks.

"Ummm," I begin as I sit up slowly, waiting for a headache to hit me or some other pain in my back to occur. "I actually feel pretty good."

"I was about to walk across the street to the market and get a snack for dad and some coffee for the morning. Do you want me to get you anything?"

I think about it for a moment, the Marina Market does have a good selection of Ben & Jerry's and I have just had a major medical procedure. I mean of all the times in your life when "calories don't count," having the fluid that protects your brain and spinal column sucked out of your back would probably be one.

"Actually, yeah, I'll have a pint of..." I start to say when the smell of the ocean wind drifts in through my living room window and gives me pause. I feel a sense of claustrophobia, like I've been trapped on my couch, not just by the procedure but by the disease itself and I see a glimpse of my future that I don't want to see. A future where I can't move. Where I am stuck inside while someone else has to wait on me hand and foot. "You know what? I'll come with you. I need to get out of here."

"Are you sure?" my dad asks. "Dr. Chan said you needed to be on your back for at least eight hours."

"It's been almost seven and I'll come right back and lie down and probably go to bed for the rest of the night anyway."

My parents look at each other in the way parents do when they're deciding who gets to be the bad cop and punish the kid, but I give them the I-probably-have-an-incurable-disease-smile and neither of them says a word. A few minutes later my mom and I cross Via Marina and start to walk the aisles of the store, picking up little items here and there to fill my cupboards back home. I glance into the freezer, ready to claim my reward for getting poked, but truthfully none of the frozen pints look that appealing. Free calories or not, Chubby Hubby is not going to be the one who can comfort me in this moment. Because while I have made it through the procedure, it is beginning to occur to me that I still have to wait for the results. Results that may or may not be confusing. If it is positive, I have MS; if it's negative, I could still have MS. Instead of ice cream, I settle on a Tootsie Pop as my prize and we head back home. Sixty-two licks later I am in my pajamas and ready for bed.

The next morning I wake up feeling great. There is no tenderness in my back and no headache. Perhaps Dr. Chan was right and I really am going to be fine.

Or perhaps Dr. Chan is a sadomasochist.

Because about five hours after I wake the headaches begin. I am at lunch with my parents and think it is probably just a latent pain that a little caffeine can cure, so I order a Coke and a hot fudge brownie sundae for dessert.

But when that doesn't work we go home and I immediately lie down on the couch. The headache is relieved and I feel good again. Maybe I had pushed myself a little too soon and my parents suggest that I take the rest of the day to hang out on my back and watch movies.

However, every time I get up to go to the bathroom the headaches return and each time I move they come back with an even stronger vengeance.

It feels like a hangover on crack. As if last night I drank three bottles of red wine, half a bottle of Popov vodka, a 12-pack of Hefeweizen, a few Zimas, and topped it all off with a box of Chardonnay before I went to bed and somehow survived to wake up the next morning.

My head is pounding and my stomach is churning. I'm nauseated from the pain. I want to die. And thanks to Google I know why it hurts so bad. The fluid that runs through my spinal sac and all the way up to my head is slowly draining and my brain is literally banging against the inside of my skull.

Of course, me being the medically obsessed girl that I am, I decide to turn this whole thing into an experiment. How long can I stay sitting up straight before the massive headache kicks in?

I use my watch like a countdown clock to birth.

I start counting the time between sitting up and the rush of pain as if I were having contractions.

Oh, I'm only at eight minutes. Not ready for a hospital yet.

Five minutes. Man that's getting painful.

Four and a half. I'm cursing that man who did this to me, but I can keep going.

Three. Just keep breathing.

One and a half. Give me the drugs.

One. Fucking A.

Thirty seconds. If you don't fix this now everyone is going to hear me scream.

And that's when my mom decides it is time to take me to the hospital.

Well, almost.

As much as I'd like to tell you that the three of us ran out to my dad's rented minivan and sped off to the hospital, we didn't. Why? Because it's a Saturday night and everyone knows those are the busiest times in a hospital. Do you know how many people get shot, stabbed, high, and drunk on a Saturday? Me neither. But apparently enough to make it not quite time to rush me to the ER.

"We're really not going to go?" my mom asks my dad.

"It's eleven on a Saturday night. We're going to end up waiting there until five or six in the morning. Wouldn't it be better to wake up early and go then?"

I think for a minute about protesting, but change my mind. "He has a point," I say, remembering the last time I went to the ER when I had an asthma attack right after college. I was stuck waiting in some horrible room by myself while some guy got handcuffed, another woman pissed her pants, and some kid kept coughing all over me. "Mom, it'll be fine. As soon as I lay down the headache goes away, I'll just go to sleep and you guys can wake me up early. Besides, maybe it'll get better."

"Are you sure you can wait until the morning? We can take you now," my mom pleads.

"I'm sure," I say. Not only do I not want to spend the night in a crowded waiting room, but doctors aren't on my list of people I want to see in the near future. After all, it was Dr. Chan who did this to me in the first place.

The next morning when I wake to use the restroom, the recurrence of the headache seems to be better. In the time it takes to get to the bathroom, pee, and get back to bed there is no sign of my brain pounding on my skull.

Once my mom hears me walking around she comes into my room.

"How are you feeling?" she asks gently.

"Good. I think it may have fixed itself," I reply. "I don't really have a headache."

"Do you want some breakfast? I cut up fruit."

When I get to the kitchen area, my dad is already at the table drinking his coffee.

"Morning," he says.

"Morning," I reply, then take one look at his outfit—shorts, leather belt, polo shirt—and know exactly what his plans for the day are.

"Are you going to play golf?" I ask.

"Ummm," he starts. "The guys out at Rancho want me to come play before work tomorrow. But you know I'll stay if you want me to. How are you feeling?"

"I'm fine actually. Don't worry. You should go play. Tell the guys I said hi."

To be fair to my dad, the reason he and my mom were able to come out to LA on such short notice was that they could turn it into a business trip, and I was supposed to be fine after Friday, so I'm not that mad. Besides, I'm feeling good and I have my mom.

After my dad leaves for the Inland Empire, which is about 45 minutes east of where I live, my mom and I start doing a little work around my apartment.

However, after a couple hours my headaches start to return.

"Mom, I don't feel so good," I say as I lay down on the couch.

"Do you think we should go to the hospital?" she asks without hesitation and I make a painful nod yes.

Half an hour later my mom and I are in a screened off room in the ER of Saint John's in Santa Monica. Apparently, a spinal fluid leak is kind of a big deal and when the intake nurses hear what happened they immediately give you a bed so you won't have to sit in the waiting room amongst infectious lepers and the like.

Inside the room my mom helps me put on one of those lovely hospital gowns that barely ties in the back and I settle onto the bed so that my headache can start to subside. After about ten minutes, a very attractive doctor in his early or mid forties enters the room. His balding/shaved head makes him look distinguished and tough, especially since I can see his biceps popping out from under his scrubs. Even though my experiences with doctors as of late hasn't been stellar, I still smile at him with my pale, makeup-less face. Maybe something good can come from this trip.

"I hear you're in pain," he says softly, and I want to say yes, please help me strong doctor—but when he turns to my mom and says, "And you're her sister?" I roll my eyes back into my pain-riddled head.

"No, I'm her mom," my mother answers with a courteous smile and a flash of her left hand and its Cartier mark that she is married.

"Oh, sorry, you look so young. You guys could almost be twins."

"Yes, I know," I say, having heard this sentiment for much of my adult life and not wanting to get into it further. I get it. My mom is young. She is hot and boys think she's a MILF. But I'm in pain over here, so let's move on.

"What happened?" the attractive doctor asks.

"I had a spinal tap and now I have a pounding headache that only goes away when I lie on my back. My doctor told me if this happened I should go to the ER."

"Well, your doctor was right. But why did you have the spinal tap in the first place?"

"Because they think I have MS."

The doctor's face drops and I can see his mind turning. I know precisely what he is thinking.

"But you're so young," he says.

"I know. I'm not exactly happy about this either."

My mom puts her hand on mine then looks to the doctor, "So, can you help her? The other doctor said something about a blood patch. Does she need that?"

"Yes. I'm going to have to find an anesthesiologist to do it though."

"You can't just give it to her?" my mom asks.

"They didn't tell you what a blood patch is, did they?"

My mom and I both shake our heads no.

"Well, it's essentially an epidural, except instead of injecting a numbing agent outside of the spinal column the anesthesiologist will have to take a vial of blood from her arm and inject that into the space between her vertebrae and the spinal sac. What then happens is that a clot will form over the hole in the sac and the leak will be sealed."

My mom responds with a blank look and I know she's terrified. She's not one for needles, blood, and other bodily fluids. In fact, doctor's offices usually scare the hell out of her.

"It'll be fine, Mom. It's just like the spinal tap only instead of taking something out they're putting something in. Trust me. It wasn't that bad. And you can close your eyes."

The doctor smiles at my mom, "She's right. You can do this."

I want to smack the man. Doesn't he know that I have a great dad? One that loves my mom? Stop flirting.

"Okay. Go ahead. You can give it to her," my mom says.

"Mom, I'm not a child, you don't have to give him permission."

My mom starts to respond but before we can get into it further, the doctor interrupts us. "Okay, so I'm going to call up to labor and delivery and see if they can spare the anesthesiologist to come down and help you. Since it's Sunday there's usually only one person up there giving epidurals, so you might have to wait a little bit. But I'll do my best to get him to come down quickly," he says with confidence as he gathers his notes and makes his way out of the curtained room.

As soon as the doctor is out of earshot my mom turns to me, "He was cute."

"Mom, he was hitting on you, not me."

"No he wasn't. He saw that I'm married."

"Doesn't matter, he still tried. And besides, he's closer to your age than mine."

"I thought you liked older guys."

"I do. When they're not hitting on my mom."

"All right. One day you'll find your doctor."

"One day," I nod then excuse myself to use the restroom.

When I return, head pounding from my excursion, the anesthesiologist arrives.

"Thanks for coming down so quickly," my mom says.

"Of course," the short plump man in need of a hip replacement says as he hobbles over to the opposite side of the bed. "I only have two women in labor upstairs and I've got at least an hour before the first one's ready for her epidural."

"Well, I'm ready," I say.

"Great. I'm going to have you lie on your side with your back facing me. It's basically going to happen like your spinal tap did, only once I get this small tube inserted into your back I'm going to have to come around and take some blood from your arm. I'll then put it into the tube and you should be as good as new."

The procedure begins just as my spinal tap did. A wash of iodine, a little pinch, some numbing, another big needle in my back and then...

Buzz. Buzz.

The anesthesiologist pauses. "I'm sorry that's my pager. Let me turn it off."

He reaches into his pocket, flips a switch then returns to my back. "Okay, I'm just about ready to get the blood." He looks at my mom and says, "I'm going to need you to be my helper. With this hip, I'm not as mobile as I used to be."

I look at my mom's face and the look of fear is priceless. "You'll be okay," I say.

"You don't like blood?" the man asks.

"She made me clean up my own vomit in seventh grade because it made her gag. What do you think?"

"Cory—"

"What? It's true. But you know I still love you," I say, tube protruding from my back.

"I'm so sorry to interrupt," a mousy nurse says as she peeks her head inside the curtain of my ER space, "but we've gotten two calls already. Labor upstairs has progressed and you're needed."

"Tell them it will have to wait 15 minutes. I need to finish here," the anesthesiologist replies.

When the nurse leaves, I turn to him and ask, "What happens if you don't get there in time?"

"The woman misses her window to get an epidural and she'll have to labor without drugs."

"Oh," I respond as a sadistic thought creeps through my mind and I wonder if the woman upstairs about to give birth is the death stare lady from the ultrasound nearly six months ago. I picture her attractive husband and his beautiful eyes and I wonder if she is now screaming at some nurse for looking at him in the wrong way. Then I hope it really is her and the rest of my blood patch will take a wee bit longer than anyone expected and the poor bitchy woman will now be giving birth au naturel. Then I think karma's a bitch as the stumpy man pulls blood from my arm and asks my mom to hold the vial while he returns to my back.

"Okay, I can take that now," the short man says as he holds out his hand. The vial of dark blood drifts over my shoulders and soon makes its way into my spinal column.

As the anesthesiologist finishes the procedure I feel a release in my head.

"Is it supposed to feel like I just popped my ears on a flight to Vegas?" I ask.

"Yes. That's the pressure of the spinal fluid re-equalizing around your brain. It's a good thing." He removes the long needle from my spine and covers it with a fresh Band-Aid.

"So, that's it, she's okay now?" my mom asks.

"Well, the blood patch is still pretty invasive and she might be in some pain when you get home. I'm going to write a prescription for Vicodin and I'm also going to suggest that as soon as you get home you get into bed and stay there for the rest of the day."

"Could the leak happen again?" I ask, afraid I'll be in that painful hangover-esque state once more.

"Most likely no, but I still want you to take it easy."

"I can do that," I say as the man starts packing up his gear to head upstairs to the pregnant witches.

"Here's my cell phone number," he says, then scrawls his digits on the back of his card. "If anything goes wrong or that headache comes back, you call me right away."

When I am finally released from the hospital the hot doctor who'd hit on my mom earlier is kind enough to personally escort us out to the car. He makes sure to help me into the passenger seat and let my mom know that if we have any questions he'll be on call for the next eight hours. I guess there are perks to having a MILF for a mom.

After I get home, take my Vicodin, read a little of Chelsea Handler's book, *Are You There Vodka? It's Me, Chelsea* (which is uber-hilarious when you're fucked up by the way), pass out, and eventually wake up the next day, I get a call from the MS specialist.

The results of the spinal tap are: "Negative."

"So now what?" I ask, shocked that they weren't positive and unsure what that means in the grand scheme of things, because a negative result doesn't necessarily mean that I don't have MS.

"I'd like to keep a watch on you. Have you come back in six months and we'll see where you're at then. In the meantime, I'm sorry that you had to go to the ER, and I hope you feel better soon."

"Thanks," I reply as I slowly hang up the phone, too shaken to ask any more questions.

My whole reality starts crashing down around me. I know that this is good news, but I can't accept it.

"What'd she say?" my mom asks as she sits on my bed.

"It came back negative."

"That's great news," she exclaims with a hug, but my body hangs limp in her arms. "What's wrong?"

I shake my head. "I don't know."

"Cory, what's wrong?"

"What's wrong is that there's something wrong with me. If it's not MS, then what is it? I can't sleep at night. My limbs go numb all the time. I'm in pain. I keep forgetting things I should know. I'm tired. I'm worn out. And now I feel like it's all in my head."

"I believe you."

"Yeah, then why do I feel like this?" I ask out of desperation.

She puts her arm around me, but for some reason I don't want it. As much as I love my mom and as much as she's been there for me through every year of my life, I don't want her sympathy.

I am pissed.

Not at her. At the world. At the doctors. At this fucking disease. It's messed with my life. It's put it on hold so that I could wait and find out what? *Negative, but you still probably have MS, but there's a chance you don't.* What kind of answer is that after a year-long wait?

I might as well be dating the damn disease 'cause it's toying with me as much as any man I've ever loved has. Coming into my life, sweeping me off my feet, turning my world upside down, making me see things in ways I never have before, leading me on like it was going somewhere, like we might have a future together, but then it gets a little scared, afraid of commitment, so it flirts with other people, makes me question all my feelings and everything I believed all along. Then I start to second-guess everything, the last voice mail, the cryptic text. I try to decipher it all, make meaning out of nothing and everything. Are we together or not? Are we going to do this? For once in my life I want to be that crazy girl, the girl who leaves ten voice mails in a row, shows up at the bar where he's with his friends, follows his car, drives by his house late at night to see if he's at home, stalks him on the internet, waits for him outside of work, all in hopes of getting an answer.

But like every man before him, I get no answer.

And when my dad returns home that night, he sits me down on the couch next to him.

"Come here," he says. "Let's talk."

And I think he's going to talk to me about relationships, about learning to let go, about how to move on, about how there are other fish in the sea.

Instead, he says nothing.

He puts his arms around me, the same ones that once taught me how to change a tire and hit a ball, and lets me curl up in the nook between his armpit and chest.

I let my head rest on the soft familiarity of his shirt and for 45 minutes straight I sob uncontrollably. Tears and deep breaths become our words.

Finally I know why this is so hard.

Like every relationship I've ever had, I have no control. I will never know if or when MS will leave me, or if we'll remain together 'til death do us part. I will never know if I'll be loved every step of the way, or if something will cause that love to fail. I will never be able to predict the hard times and I am guaranteed there will be times when I cannot get out of bed.

There is one thing, however, that will remain constant.

I've known it since the day my very first crush ripped up the Valentine's card I made for him and Red Hots candies spilled out onto the floor of our school bus. I've known it since I returned home in tears and my dad threatened to walk out the door and kick that boy's butt. I've known that, no matter what, my family will always be there. And that is something I can count on forever, not a disease.

Chapter Twenty-Two

HEY LOVER

"I think I'm about to take a lover," I tell Colleen over Mexican one night, several weeks after the spinal tap.

"Really?" she asks.

"Why not?" I reply.

When I was a senior in high school, my parents sold the house we lived in and moved us to a newly constructed townhouse in the next town over. As part of the compensation for the fact that we were now a 15-minute drive to school instead of five, we were allowed to paint our rooms any color we wanted.

I chose to paint mine a brilliant red. It was a deep rich color, which I then proceeded to cover with poems I had written throughout the years. Over my door, I wrote the words *Agape, Caritas, Eros*. The three words for love. The love between God and man, the love of friendship and family, and the love of the erotic.

I thought I was clever. But more than that I wanted to experience all three of these loves in my lifetime. The first two were easy, but the third had eluded me. Until I met the Englishman.

Here's how it started: My friends and I were at my new favorite spot, the Otheroom in Venice. We'd just saddled up to the concrete bar and ordered some drinks when I heard the accent.

"What are you drinking?" an older foreigner asked me.

"A Chimay," I replied, as I brought the glass to my lips and took a sip of the smooth beer.

"I'll have one of what she's having," he told the bartender before turning to me. "It better not be any of that watered-down American crap," he said with a wink.

"Don't worry," I replied with a smile. "I know how you Englishmen are. If you don't like it, I'll buy your next drink."

The alien took a seat next to me and we began to chat. After my summer in England I knew how to work these foreigners. Let them know you're intelligent, but then play it cool like you don't have much going on except what it is you're doing right now: Drinking a beer in a dark bar trying to find a date for the following Saturday evening.

We continued to talk and soon I found out that he too was a writer. He had written a well-known blockbuster movie and was now in the states living in his manager's guesthouse. As I took a look at the Rolex on his wrist, I promptly assumed this was some fabulous place in Beverly Hills. Then I thought about his success and felt a tad bit ashamed that I hadn't done anything of significance in quite a while. Instead of writing, I had basically spent the past year and a half of my life playing medical detective and doing the work I needed to do to get by, but nothing had made its way from the synapses of my brain onto the pixels of my computer.

However, this subject was not broached in our talk. We kept it simple and breezy and because I told him I had studied at Cambridge I won him over.

When he finished the remaining sips of his beer he looked me in the eyes and said, "Well, m'lady, I think I'm done here for the night… can I get your phone number?"

"I don't know," I said. "Are you actually going to call? 'Cause I don't give my number out to every stranger I meet."

"Of course," he said as he took my hand and kissed the top of it as if I were European royalty. "I never ask and don't call."

I gave him my number and as he left I imagined him returning home to his casita and having a nightcap as he sat in the moonlight and pondered life and the world's problems. Then I imagined he and I together in the weeks to follow. The two of us sipping cocktails poolside as we basked in the Southern California sun. I, in heels, a low-cut one piece, shades, and an oversized hat, and he in topsiders and form fitting shorts. The cabana boy would feed us grapes and when it got too hot we'd dip our feet in the water then retire to his room where we'd lie naked in bed as the bamboo fan danced above us. We'd be straight out of a scene from Gatsby and we'd fall in love, or...

"For real, I think I'm about to take a lover," I tell Colleen just a week after I had met the Englishman.

"And what does that entail?" she asks.

"I don't know for sure, but I have a feeling I might like it," I smile as I remember that I had had a semi-lover once.

We were 16 and he was from Spain. We were on the family room couch when he excused himself to the kitchen and returned with a surprise.

"Do you want to play a Spanish game?" he asked.

"Sure," I smiled.

"Close your eyes," he said. I closed them and the next thing I knew there was something cold on my neck. When I blinked my eyes open, Alberto's face was thisclose to mine. I could feel the heat from his cheeks and in between his teeth was an ice cube, which he gracefully danced upon my décolletage. The cool water dripped down my skin and when the solid ice had melted to the size of a diamond he kissed me and let the remaining bits of cold drift into my mouth. Our tongues intertwined as the last sliver of ice melted between us. We went to Homecoming that fall. We held hands in the hall. It was the perfect teenage introduction to seduction. Loverville at 16. (I can only imagine what it will be like today at 29 with a man who's 43.)

"But how do you know he wants to be a lover?" Colleen asks.

"Because he keeps texting me sexy messages," I reply succinctly.

"Like dick pics?"

"No. He has a way with words."

Plus, he never calls—he only writes. And I've dated enough in LA to know that he doesn't want to truly date me, he only wants one thing.

"Okay," Colleen says with a sigh.

"Look, I think having a lover will be a good thing."

Since I found out about the MS I've been looking at every man as if he could be some sort of savior. Constantly feeling like I am living in 18th-century high society and at any moment some baron will come by, steal a giant lock of my hair, and I will no longer be desirable. By the time my hair grows back it will be too late, I'll be past my prime and there will be no man for me to marry.

But now I don't give a shit. I just want to have fun and not have to worry if he's the one.

"All I want to worry about is my outfit and my hair," I say.

"Well, cheers to that," Colleen responds, agreeing with my plan.

On our first date, I invite the Englishman to my place. I put on a short black dress and curl my hair so that it cascades around my face in long beachy waves. For foreplay, we make dinner and open a bottle of Cabernet. After the last bite, the Brit says, "come here," in a voice that makes him sound like I am a lady being awed by all of parliament. We leave the mess in the kitchen and slowly make our way to my room.

Articles of clothing fall to the floor like petals of roses, and soon we are naked in bed.

I breathe in each bit of his pale English skin that stands in stark contrast to my brightly colored sheets. He is tall and lanky and his strawberry blonde hair is beginning to recede, but his accent and demeanor have me believing he is tall, dark, and handsome.

We make love as lovers do, with no expectations for the future.

For several weeks this routine continues: dinner, wine, sex. Conversations stay breezy and there is no other talk of our careers or questions about our lives.

On our fifth date, however, we break routine and head to a local Spanish restaurant, because let's be honest, unless you're a sixpence whore, it's impossible to spend all your time doing it. There I finally tell the Englishman that I am a writer too. When he asks what I am working on, I hesitate then tell him I am writing a memoir.

"What is it about?" he asks.

"Dating in LA mostly," I say, giving him my rehearsed response so that I don't have to reveal my secret.

"Sounds unique," he says as he goes back to nibbling on his bacon-covered fig appetizer and gazes off into the distance.

I can tell that he is not impressed with my response, but who can blame him? A book about dating? Written by a single girl living in a big city? Nope, never seen that before.

"Um, it's a little more than dating stories," I begin, trying to prove I have some clout in the writing world.

"I'm sure it is," he interrupts as he finishes his Rioja in a blasé manner. "Should we order another glass or get the check?"

He motions over my shoulder for the bartender.

"I've got stories about celebrities in there too," I say out of desperation, like a little girl tugging on her dad's pant legs. *Notice me. Notice me.*

"Uh, huh."

The bartender arrives and he orders another round.

"And I kissed a girl once."

"You do remember that I'm European, right?"

"Yeah," I say, knowing full well that that means he's probably seen and experienced far more sexually deviant acts than a drunken co-ed kissing her sorority sister.

"Don't worry, I'm sure your book will sell someday," he says completely patronizing me. "You're cute, publishers like that."

"Excuse me?"

"I'm kidding."

But it doesn't feel like he's kidding, and I now want to defend my work. Instead, I take a long sip of my Albarino and remind myself: *His opinion does not matter. This man is just a lover. What do I care?*

But I do. As much as I'd played it cool when I'd first met the foreigner, I don't want him to think I'm a complete idiot.

"Finish that," he says as the bartender brings us our last round.

I take one look at him in his condescending sport coat and chug the remaining ounces of wine. Then I open my mouth and let it go.

"I lied. My book's not about dating. I have multiple sclerosis," I say. His face drops. "So I've been writing about my experiences with that, doctors, dating, dealing. Just so you know."

Without a word, he sets his glass on the wooden bar and looks at me. I prepare myself for the worst. Any minute now I am sure he will ask for the check, hail us a cab, drop me at home, and never call again.

However, something completely unexpected happens.

"But you look so healthy. And you seem so calm," he says as he grabs my hand.

"I am pretty healthy. I've also had time to process it all."

"I had no clue," he says.

"Most people don't. Truthfully, it usually takes me a long time to tell anyone."

"Well, I'm glad you told me."

"You are?"

"Of course," he says, pulling me in close to him.

I let my head rest on his chest as I take a deep breath in.

"And so you know," he begins, "this doesn't change my perspective of you one bit. In fact, this only makes me think you're more amazing than I already thought."

"Thanks," I say.

"And I'm here if you need anything."

"Really?"

He nods yes and I think, *Who is this man? What happened to my lover? The man who was there for sex, not emotional support?*

When we arrive back to my apartment we open a bottle of champagne and sit on my patio. It is a cool November evening so we wrap ourselves in blankets and talk as the air becomes foggy. Halfway through the bottle of bubbly our conversation turns to the serious, my life and my disease.

"You must be scared," he says.

"I am," I reply, and without warning my eyes well with tears.

Of all the friends and family who have been there for me over the past year, this is the first time someone has come out and acknowledged my fear. Soon my cheeks are flooded and stained with everything I've been holding inside. He holds me as I cry then says, "Let's go. I want to show you something." He helps me stand up then leads me into my bedroom where he places me on the bed with a slow embrace.

Then he gathers up my laptop, types in a few things, and before I know it I am watching Warren Zevon's last interview with David Letterman.

A man who is dying is talking about death.

I hang on to each and every word as if it is a life raft sent down from above.

Even though I know I am not dying, there is something about my situation that feels fatal. Like: If everything the doctors say comes true a real part of me will die.

When the interview is over, we watch the singer's entire last performance. The sentiments of his songs whisper in my heart as the Englishman and I dance in the room.

When the songs slow and the final one plays, we lie on my bed watching Warren sing the last words of his life and I contemplate the fact that the foreigner's reaction to my situation is what I've been searching for over the past year.

Only it has come in the form of a lover, someone I had no intention of having real feelings for.

Having a lover was supposed to be different. We were supposed to have illicit sex in foreign places on Frette sheets. Conjugate in a guesthouse in Beverly Hills. Sip cocktails and frolic in an infinity pool. Limit our talks to sweet nothings and the weather. Then one day when we'd had enough caressing, when we'd had our fill of each other, we'd calmly walk away with no regrets and no reason to return. We'd forget each other's names and go back to our lives. Our time together would simply be a memory, an easy sketch of a romanticized notion of carefree lovemaking.

But now, in my room as the Englishman and I listen to Warren Zevon, I begin to rethink my plan.

In the weeks that follow our second date of staying up until the sun blossomed, I consistently think about this question: *Am I a fool to allow him to remain just a lover? Or should I look for more?*

I continue to see the Englishman as a way to test the water. We see each other once or twice a week for weeks on end. We go out on fancy dates. We go to Hollywood parties and talk to famous writers. All of this is great, but yet I wade with apprehension. That is until it happens. The moment that seals it all.

It is a typical date, much like our first. We've uncorked a bottle of Sauvignon Blanc and are sipping away on my couch. As we talk, the light of the moon drifts into my living room and the gentle ocean breeze raps at the window.

The wine has settled into my body and I am feeling quite tipsy. And, I might add, quite romantic. I lean over and kiss my Englishman, gently toying with his lips. He laughs and kisses me back as our hands explore each other's bodies. Soon things become heated, and he whispers, "I have an idea."

He directs me to go into the bedroom and wait for him. I prop myself up on the bed, lean my head into my arm and allow my hair to gently fall down my back.

Finally, he enters the room with one of my dining room chairs and my laptop. Without a word, he sets the chair down in the empty space between my bed and the mirrored closet doors. Then he places the computer on top of my dresser and searches through iTunes until he finds exactly what he is looking for. He hits play and as the slow moving sounds of "Purple Rain" fill the air, he seats himself in the wooden upright chair then looks to me.

"I want you to dance," he says.

I take one look at him and laugh. "You're joking, right?"

He shakes his head. "No."

"Really?" I ask.

"Please? Pretty please."

"Fine," I say as I get up off the bed, stand in front of him and move my hips side to side in a fairly robotic fashion. "There."

"Oh, come on," he says as he places his hands on my hips and tries to guide them into seduction. "I know you can do better than that."

He's right. I probably can. I took plenty of dance classes as a kid, was a cheerleader in high school, have great rhythm, and thanks to yoga can still do the splits. But standing in front of him I feel small and shy like a young child being put on the spot and asked to perform her latest recital piece for the entire family, creepy uncles included.

"I can't," I say.

"Sure you can."

"I feel silly."

"Don't. You're beautiful." He gently guides me onto his lap. "Just feel the music."

As I straddle him in the chair, he pulls me in for a kiss. Our lips meet and our tongues dance between us.

Soon one song bleeds into the next and I start to recall all the strippers I have seen in the past. Slowly, our bodies start to move to the beat of the music. I feel a surge of confidence and soon I am channeling my inner Demi Moore. My body moves in one fluid motion and I playfully dance all around him.

I slowly and seductively discard my clothes until I am left wearing nothing but Victoria's best secret. My Englishman gets more and more turned on, but I gently remind him of the house rules, "no touching."

While I am lacking the Lucite heels and baby powder scent, I surely could be the big breadwinner if this were amateur night down at Crazy Girls.

After a while, I can tell he wants the session to be over. Not because he's had enough of me, but because he can't get with me. However, what he doesn't realize is that this is no longer about playful foreplay.

This has turned into a whole other animal.

Watching his face twist in frustration, as he is restricted from touching me, I feel a sense of power. Being able to use my body in such a commanding way that I can practically make a man cry is empowering. As the music continues on, I continue to dance. Harder, faster, more seductively. I swivel, sway, and contort my hips and legs in ways I never have before. Endorphins rush through my blood and a euphoric sense of ease comes over me.

The dance has set me free.

Like Sleeping Beauty and the kiss of her prince, it is the Englishman's request that has awoken me from my slumber. My body has been reclaimed from the wrath of disease and no one can take that away from me now. No doctor. No test. No well-meaning friend. No one.

For weeks after this night, the Englishman and I become inseparable. We spend a lot of time at my place, sipping wine, making love, talking, and—most importantly—dancing.

But there is one problem.

I am so wrapped up in how I feel, how I perceive him, that I have yet to stop and ponder anything about him.

So I begin to ask:

"It's silly your manager is always dropping you off here. Why don't you let me give you a ride?"

Even though it is December, I still want to sit by the pool and sip cocktails and let the pool boy wait on us hand and foot.

He continuously pushes off my requests, saying that he doesn't mind coming to my place, but finally, on a Friday, I get my wish.

"My manager's going out of town for the night," he starts, "so I've got to stay for a little bit and let the dog out, but if you want to come over here you can. Then we can go out and do whatever you want."

"Okay," I say. "Text me the address."

I sit in anticipation, waiting to find out where this amazing home is going to be. But when the text comes through I am instantly disappointed.

The zip code does not point to Beverly Hills. It clearly spells out that it is over the hill and, well, far away.

It is in the Valley.

Ughh, I think. Princes are supposed to live in castles on hills, not shacks in low-lying plains, far away from the hustle of Los Angeles. But I stop myself from being completely superficial and remember that there are plenty of nice neighborhoods in the Valley with plenty of room for infinity pools and casitas.

At six o'clock I hop in my car and head to his place. After sitting in nearly two hours of traffic I pull up to the house. In the dark everything looks fine, but when the neighbor across the way opens her front door the light from inside bathes her yard in truth.

We are no longer in the glamour of LA. We might as well be back in Kansas.

The homes on the street are small and rundown and the front yards are overgrown with weeds and protected by chain link fences. I double-check the address just to be sure I am in the right place.

The neighbor across the way shuts her door and the street goes dark again. I park my car in front of the house and steel myself with a fresh coat of M.A.C. Lipglass. If I'm not going to be fanned by a pool boy the least I can do is look pretty.

When I get to the front door of the house, I hear an accent call my name.

"I'm back here. Come around through the carport."

I walk to the side of the house under what I'm assuming is a carport though there are no cars and the wood above me appears as if it would collapse with any movement over a one on the Richter scale.

"Hello, sexy," he says as he pulls me in close.

"Hi," I reply, reluctantly returning his kiss. "So this is where you live, huh?"

"This is it," he says proudly. "Want to see the guesthouse?"

"Sure." *Frette, Frette, Frette, there better be Frette.*

He leads me by the hand to a door on the side of a small structure in the backyard, then opens it. Upon sight, I immediately freeze. This is no guesthouse. This is half of an old garage converted into a room. A room with a worn down couch, a desk, and an air mattress on the floor.

"Well, don't just stand there, come on in."

I gently step inside, my feet heavy below me. The floor may be carpeted but clearly it is pure concrete underneath.

"This is nice," I mutter.

But it isn't nice. Not for the fact that it isn't made of marble or perched next to water. It isn't nice because it isn't what I had envisioned. This is not the image of the man who'd set me free. This is a man who is lost.

"I need to walk the dog, but then we can go wherever you want. There're a few great bars around here or we could head back towards your place. It's up to you."

"Let's go back to Venice," I reply. I want to go back to my safe normal neighborhood, where the man at the bar has a distinguished accent and a real career.

When we get back to Venice I drive us straight to Abbot Kinney with the intention that the Englishman will buy me enough drinks at the Otheroom that everything I've seen in the Valley will dissipate into a mirage. Then after, we'll go home and I'll dance again, showing him some new moves I've dreamt up. Unfortunately, the line to get in has more than 20 people, and there is no way I am waiting for intoxication.

"Let's go across the street," I suggest half seriously and half to see his reaction. The place across the way is the only gay bar in the area and I am hoping to give him a chance to redeem himself. If he is confident enough in his manhood and tolerant enough of other's expression of their sexuality, then I'm a fool to judge him based on the fact that he is a little down on his luck at the moment.

"Sure, sounds fun," he says.

Inside, the bar is full of men. Handsome ones, muscular ones, older ones, and pretty ones.

"What do you want?" he asks.

"Vodka soda," I reply, heading straight for the quick buzz, not a slow wine- or beer-induced one.

He orders a scotch on the rocks and when the bartender returns with our drinks, he looks to me, "Uh, can you get this one? I don't have any cash."

I start to protest, but then see the sign above the bar: CASH ONLY. I give him the benefit of the doubt: It isn't that he doesn't want to pay, it's that he literally can't.

I pay the bill and take a seat at the bar. My Englishman excuses himself to the bathroom and I soon find myself in a conversation with a nice older gentleman. He's been living in Venice for the past 30 years and loves how tolerant the area is. I agree. The place is great. He then proceeds to give me an oral history of the entire city by the sea. I get so enthralled in his story that I fail to notice that my Englishman has yet to return from the bathroom.

At one point I look over and see him chatting with a guy at the jukebox. That's nice, I think, he's making friends.

But another 15 minutes passes by and soon my new friend is tapping me on the shoulder.

"Oh, look at your friend. That's sweet."

"He's not my friend, he's my boyfr—"

OH. MY. GOD. My man is kissing another man.

I nearly choke on my vodka at the site of the Englishman frenching the hot dude in the corner. Is he cheating on me?

I mean your guy's not supposed to kiss someone else. But does it count if it's another guy?

If it were any place else I probably would have stormed off, but now I can't. I am in a gay bar and I don't want to cause a scene because I don't want to look like the intolerant asshole from the Midwest.

I am screwed. Especially when the Englishman brings over his new friend and introduces me to him.

"Cory, meet John."

"Your friend's a really good kisser," the other man says as he shakes my hand. "And he's got a nice accent too."

"I do, don't I?" the Englishman says as the hot guy kisses him again.

What the hell is happening? I know Europeans are supposed to be open with their sexuality, but this is just confusing.

Does he like me? Does he like him? Is he into men or women or both?

Shit, this is worse than trying to decipher whether to stick with a man who's lied about where he's living and how successful he really is. This is a whole pile of craziness that I have no clue how to handle. So I do the only thing I can think of.

Nothing.

I smile politely and laugh at how cute the Englishman and his new friend are together. Then I go home. Alone. Two days later I leave for Christmas vacation with my family, figuring it will work out on its own.

And it does: At the core of it all, the Englishman cheated on me and I am not going to stand for it.

So when I return to LA after the holidays I end things with him.

"I'm sorry, I don't think this is going to work."

I expect him to understand and handle things in a mature way, but instead he hangs up on me, and a week later I get this text message:

Despite your MS, when everyone (oh yes, I told them—I wanted some advice) told me I was fucking insane to be with you, I would have married you ... Everyone tells me I've dodged the bullet and that I have the opportunity to find a healthy, loving partner and mother for my kids, who might actually stay alive to see them grow ... Remember: when you're fucking some guy ... and you tell him about the MS—you can kiss good-bye to ever seeing him again!

And that's the last I ever hear from the Englishman. Every now and then I check the trades to see if he's sold a script, but there's never been a word about him. For all I know he's been deported, and that's fine by me.

Chapter Twenty-Three

A SIGN FROM ABOVE

Sometimes you have to go dark. And I don't mean shady shit, like hanging out in back alleys and smoking crack, I mean you have to lay low, stay away from bars, and, more importantly, stop dating. This is what I did after the Englishman.

After his words showed up on my phone, I decided it was time to take a break from men. Instead I focused on work and my health. I went back to writing and I committed myself to a daily yoga practice. Slowly the depression that had seeped in and kept me slumbering through most of my days lifted and for nearly eight months I went back to living a somewhat normal life. But soon I found myself dealing with the MS once again.

I have always been a meticulous, anal retentive, speller.

In seventh grade, I was bored by every spelling list we ever had. In order to make spelling more challenging, I would sit at my desk and think about the next word. I would concentrate really hard on what I wanted it to be and most of the times my teacher would say it.

"*Example.* Jesus is an example of a martyr. *Example.*"

He'd then repeat the spelling word once more. But by that point I had already moved on to the next word on the test. *Superstitious.* I wrote the word on my paper and waited for him to call it out. "Superstitious," he said.

The other kids wrote furiously as I sat back and smiled and started to concentrate on the next word. My control over the spelling tests got better and better as the year progressed, and by the time I hit eighth grade, I was so confident in my ability to predict the spelling words that I'd finish my test before the teacher had finished reading out all the words.

Now, I'm sure there is some statistic or equation of probability that would explain why I was able to predict my spelling test words before they were even said, but that's not the point. The point is I am really good at spelling and those tests bored the hell out of me so I had to make up games of my own in order to be challenged. In fact, there is only one time I can remember where I have completely messed up.

At 12 years old I lost the county spelling bee on the word *rhetoric*. I can still remember leaving out the "h." *Retoric,* printed as I spelled it then, was the last mistake I ever made. The word was unfamiliar to me at the time. Now it is ingrained in my head. Since that loss I have been determined to spell everything correctly. In college, my papers, whether they were good or not, were always without spelling error. This attention to detail was something I took pride in.

In fact, during my first job in Hollywood, my boss discovered this talent of mine and exploited it to the best of her ability. I was tasked with proofing every document she created before she sent it out to directors, producers, and heads of studios. She offered up my services as an editor to the screenwriters whose scripts our company was paying hundreds of thousands of dollars for. I read through their work with a red pen and was praised for my ability to spot all of the errors.

I thought this talent of mine would never falter. Unfortunately, this is no longer the case.

My writing is now riddled with mistakes.

What used to take minutes, what used to roll from my head through my fingers to the keyboard on my Mac in an effortless way is now a jumbled mess.

Sentences in my work should appear as so: *In a crescent shaped valley surrounded by cliffs, there exists a haunted forest where only the tops of the trees are green and luscious, but below that, the trees are grey and deformed.*

Instead, they appear on screen like this: *In a crescent shaded valley surrounded by cliffs, their exists a haunted forest where only the tons of the trees are grapes and luscious, but below that, the teas are grey and defecated.*

The words are not misspelled. The punctuation is not wrong. But the use of the incorrect words shows that my brain has skipped a beat and wandered to a different story. When I see this on screen I start to panic. I have a way of covering my memory loss and inability to find the right words when I'm out with friends or talking to others, but I can't drink a glass of wine every time I have to work. So I go back to playing medical detective online and I learn that MS patients can develop what they call *cog fog*. It is essentially cognitive difficulties and, like every other part of this disease, manifests in everyone differently. It can be as simple as talking more slowly or losing your train of thought, or it can get as bad as misunderstanding conversations, using incorrect words, or slurring your speech. The degree of the cognitive disruption directly correlates to the amount of lesions on the brain. The more you have, the worse off you are.

I have five.

This translates for me into extra work. Into extra time spent going over the writing I do, re-writing the sentences I carefully craft in my head, looking at my prose again and again. It is my way of coping.

It's a repetitive mess that never stops.

So I rewrite and I rewrite until it appears to those who are reading that there is nothing wrong with me. I become so intent on hiding any effects of the disease that I literally write them out of existence.

And for a while, over a year in fact, this works and I am able to pretend that the MS has not severely affected my life.

But then the news comes.

December 7, 2010.

I am sitting at my computer, scrolling through various sites, researching plot lines for my bosses, when I discover that Elizabeth Edwards has passed away.

I immediately burst into tears.

Though we had only met briefly, it is her story that has brought me back to my story. And now it is clear, everything I thought, every fear I had, has finally come true.

It is all over the news. Five o'clock. Eleven o'clock. Gawker. The Huffington Post.

John Edwards cheated on his wife and fathered a child with the other woman. The relationship and the heir were kept secret. While an ailing Elizabeth stood by her husband's side in his political pursuits, he had gone astray. His story of infidelity came out just months before her passing. He would eventually go to trial because they speculated that he had used campaign funds to support his affair, but that did not stop my own speculating. Was her illness the reason for the betrayal? Or would it have happened regardless of the situation? On the day that I met her, her optimism to fight the disease was palpable, but now I know that it had dwindled.

I used to look up to that man, Mr. Presidential Hopeful. The man who stood by the side of his wife as she stood by the side of him. It was a relationship I wanted, or so I thought. But now he is a different man, and the singular nagging question that popped into my head at the beginning of all this, *Who's going to marry me now?*, is being broadcast throughout the world. The answer is out there. There is no room left to wonder. The Englishman had put it into words. A digital rendering of my every worry, an honest response. "No one," he replied.

The sentiment echoes through the senator's actions.

I post to my Facebook wall, "Sometimes one person comes into your life and has more impact than they'll ever know. Prayers to the Edwards family." It is not meant for anyone to understand or for anyone to comment upon. It is a post in solidarity to a woman who was suffering in love and in health, because while my story may not be the exact same as hers, I understand.

Though I've tried hard to forget what the Englishman said, immersing myself in writing and yoga, his words continue to pop up in my head. "You. Dead. Dying."

I do my best to carry on, but this is not always easy, which is why I have called my friends. I cannot sit at home alone.

At one of our favorite Santa Monica bars, we chat about the day's events. The passing of a caring woman and the horrific actions of men. It is not a sob story, but a way to vent and connect as girls.

And when a guy comes up behind me and orders a drink I ignore him. But this turns out to be the wrong thing to do, as I have forgotten that every guy likes a challenge.

"You girls having fun tonight?" the guy asks as soon as he receives his glass of liquid courage from the bartender.

My friends all smile politely and nod, yes. I continue to keep my back to the guy as I nod along with my friends. I expect him to leave, but he apparently takes this as an invitation to take the conversation further.

He taps me on the back and says, "You're pretty quiet. What's your name?"

I glance over my shoulder and quickly say, "Cory."

"I'm Ryan," he replies as he extends his hand, forcing me to turn my chair all the way around to face him. "Nice to meet you."

His handshake is strong and he looks me straight in the eyes.

"Nice to meet you too," I say softly.

Our palms linger together for a few more seconds before we both let go.

"What brings you out tonight?" he casually asks.

"You know. Girls' night," I say, hoping he'll get the hint.

"Oh," he says with a disappointed look. "I'm sorry for interrupting."

"No, no, it's okay," I instinctively reply, not wanting to hurt his feelings, but still hoping he'll leave.

"You sure?"

No, but I'm a nice girl so…

"Yeah, it's fine," I say.

"What do you do?" he asks.

I hesitate, then reply, "I'm a writer."

"What kind?"

"I used to work in TV," I say, "but now I'm working on a book."

He nods in the way that most people in LA do when they think you're just another girl who left the Midwest to follow her dreams in the big city and I figure he'll be done talking to me at any moment.

"What's it about?" he asks.

I think about giving him my normal spiel:

I'm writing about dating in LA and the men I meet here so you better be good or you just might end up in my book.

But with Ryan, I think, *Screw it.* I can see right through his tactics and I know he is just trying to get my number or get me into bed and I am not interested. Plus, I just want to be with my friends. So I decide to throw it all out there and see how fast he'll run.

"Well, I don't normally tell people this, but the truth is my doctors say I have multiple sclerosis. It's been a pretty rough time dealing with all the tests and the uncertainty of it all, so I'm writing about my experiences."

Ryan sits quiet for a moment and I am certain he is planning his exit strategy: "Oh look at the time, I got to go," or "My mom just called I need to go outside and call her back." But none of these excuses come out of his mouth.

Instead, all he says is, "Really? My dad has MS."

Suddenly, I am the one who is silenced. Usually this conversation, if I even have it at all, is about me, but now it is about someone else and I am dumbfounded. I have forgotten that there are others out there who are in my same situation. Somehow I've convinced myself that these people exist in some other ether, not in a place where I might meet them or their families in person.

"I'm sorry to hear that," I finally utter.

"It's okay. I guess I should've said, *'had* MS.' He doesn't have it anymore."

"You mean they thought he had it but it was something else?" I ask, knowing full well that there is no cure, but that doctors sometimes make mistakes, especially with a disease that's so difficult to diagnose.

"No. He had it. Thirty years ago he was in a wheelchair, but he refused to accept his fate. So he did a lot of research and got into holistic medicine and started to believe in mind over matter and now he's completely fine."

Despite the fact that the dark bar is packed and my friends are sitting just two feet away, I feel the entire room get silent, as if Ryan has shown me some sort of holy grail.

In all my research on the internet and all my appointments with the doctors, I have never heard a story like this.

"Are you serious?" I ask.

"Yeah. A lot of doctors have studied my dad and there have been many papers and books published on his case."

"That's amazing," I say, still in awe.

"I know. You just need to keep a positive attitude. Which, and I know I've only known you for about 20 minutes or so, it seems like you already do."

"I try," I say.

"I think you're going to be fine," Ryan replies as he gently places his hand over mine, reassuring me that he meant what he said.

"I don't mean to sound forward, but would you mind if I got your number?" Ryan asks.

I hesitate for a moment then say, "Not at all."

Even though I've had bad luck with men in bars, I feel like this is some sort of cosmic intervention and I'd be a fool to ignore it. If Ryan's dad cured himself, then certainly I can find a way to cure myself and maybe Ryan can help.

He hands over his phone and I program my number into it.

When I return home that night, alone, I sit on the couch and think about fate and the universe and how sometimes the right people show up in your life at the right time for all the right reasons and maybe men aren't so evil after all. And just as I have that thought my phone buzzes. It is a number I don't know. I pick it up in case it is one of my friends calling from somewhere else, needing me to come get them; but it isn't a friend, it's Ryan.

"Hey," he starts. "I know this might sound weird, but I really enjoyed talking to you tonight and I kind of don't want it to end. Would It be okay if I came over and we hung out?"

Despite the fact that I can hear my mother's voice screaming in my head, *Don't invite strangers over late at night, especially men you meet at bars,* I say, "sure," and give Ryan my address.

Twenty minutes later we are on my couch making small talk. It feels so natural and right that maybe all of this was meant to be and everything will work out in the end. Without even realizing what I am doing I start to fantasize about our future. We'll date, I'll meet his parents, his dad will teach me his tricks, and I'll be cured.

But there is one problem with this fantasy.

And I find it out when he kisses me.

"I have a girlfriend," he says. "I'm sorry, but I can't do this."

As I sit stunned on my couch, Ryan quietly leaves my place and I never hear from him again.

Weeks later, I tried to search for his dad and the papers written about him, but Ryan never gave me his dad's name, nor his last name and I came up empty-handed.

Perhaps he lied about the whole thing, or perhaps he was telling the truth, either way I have learned my lesson.

That night, as I slumber and drift into REM, I find myself being chased in a nightmare. But instead of succumbing to the threat behind, I start to fly. I kick my legs in one fell swoop as if I were swimming butterfly and circle my arms out and around, gliding further and further from danger. Up and up, away and away. This is how my body works when I sleep. If ever I find myself in trouble I can always fly. It is a technique I have practiced since my days as a young dreamer. It is a power I wish I possessed in my waking life. That when things got too rough or scary or dangerous I could simply flutter my feet and fly away.

Chapter Twenty-Four

SHIT HAPPENS

Today I shit my pants. One week ago I woke up and couldn't walk.

It's a beautiful life I lead, a combo of MS, a torn meniscus, and the bowel-moving effects of painkillers. I know you're totally jealous and thinking, *God, I want to be like her.* But don't worry, we can all crap our drawers if we put our minds to it. You just need to clear your head, take a couple of deep breaths, and think positive thoughts—a method I've learned through yoga known as the power of intention and making shit happen.

Which is exactly what I did. Here's how:

An old soccer injury had finally taken its toll on my left knee and I'd had surgery seven days prior to this May day. The doctors had removed a piece of cartilage from my knee and sent me on my way. For two days I laid on my couch doing nothing, downing Percocet like it was water, and icing my knee like it was the last iceberg on the planet and I couldn't let it melt. When the pain subsided I began to move around. Soon, no longer on crutches, I decide that I want to get out of my apartment for lunch, even though I am not the most mobile.

I am on the return trip, barely over half a block from my apartment when the rumbling in my bowels begins.

"Uh, oh," I say to my younger sister, Cassie, who is accompanying me on my first outing since my power to walk has been compromised.

"Are you okay?" she asks.

I think about my options—car, taxi, duck behind a bush—as the rumbling turns into painful cramping.

"There's no time," I say.

"What is wrong with you?" my sister panics. "Should I call a doctor?" Even though I'd only had a simple surgery, I know that my sister is thinking the worst. That whatever pain I am having isn't caused by my recent procedure, but the MS. It is hard not to think that way. I do my best not to, but my sister, who only recently moved out to Los Angeles with her boyfriend, hasn't spent much time with me in the last two years and so I know that has to be on her mind.

"No." I flex the muscles of my ass and press my cheeks together. "I don't need a doctor."

"Then why do you look like you're in pain?"

"I have to go to the bathroom," I say in desperation, grabbing my gut and scrunching my face.

"Oh God, gross. It's not number one, is it?" she asks, as she realizes what is happening. I shake my head in concurrence. "Then walk faster," she says.

I try to pick up the pace but my left leg is locked and barely bending. Earlier that afternoon, it had taken me nearly 30 minutes just to get to the cafe two and a half blocks from my place. Now I need to get home in less than three minutes and the fact that I've been out and about for the last two hours is not helping my situation.

"Can you hold it?" my sister asks.

"I don't think so," I say as I start to waddle like a duck in an attempt to keep moving.

"Maybe you could go a little faster."

She walks behind me as if she was rounding me up for a cattle call and I try to move quicker, but my leg is throbbing and my behind is starting to burn.

"Are you squeezing your butt cheeks together?"

I reflexively squeeze them even harder, the same way I contract my vaginal muscles as soon as someone mentions the word *Kegels*.

"What else am I supposed to do?"

"I don't know. At least you look good in those pants. Are they Lululemon?"

"Yes, but they're not going to look good for much longer."

My sister, a mirror image of me at five four with blonde hair and a sizable chest, starts laughing.

"It's not funny," I say. "Help me."

"What do you want me to do? I'm not carrying you. What if you poop on me?"

"I'm not going to poop on you. Just come here," I demand as I point to a flat spot on the sidewalk in front of me. "Let me grab on to your shoulders and you can drag me."

"Fine. But if you—"

"I'm not going to."

She gets in front of me and I wrap my arms around her upper back, but when she starts to walk we barely move.

"Use your legs," she says.

"I can't."

"Why not?"

"Because I'm holding them together so it doesn't come out."

"Oh, God," she says, and quickly squeezes out of my grip.

"Ouch," I scream. Her sudden movement had forced me to put more pressure on my leg than I'd intended and the pain soars up my thigh.

Tears form in my eyes.

"Don't cry, we're getting close," she says.

"I know. I know. But it hurts and I'm an adult and what if someone drives by and sees me and there's feces dripping down my leg?"

My sister looks around for a minute searching for options. Then she makes an observation, "I could get you one of those poop bags from over there."

My giant apartment complex allows pets, so stationed around the grounds are tall dispensers of bags to encourage owners to clean up after their dogs.

"I'm not shitting in a bag."

"Then give me your keys."

"What are you going to do? Run away and leave me out here?"

"No," she begins. "I'm going to run ahead of you, open all the doors, and hold the elevator so that you won't have to wait for it."

"Good idea."

My sister takes off running and I do my best to move as fast as I can in my condition, but I am walking at about the same pace as an Olympic runner six feet under.

I keep my legs clenched together and do my best to keep all I'd eaten over the last day inside, but my efforts are becoming more and more futile and I know I'll soon reach a point where the muscles in my lower regions will give way to an inevitable mud slide.

Tears pool in my eyes from the pain in my knee, and I fantasize about taking another Percocet and falling fast asleep under its influence, but I keep going.

Finally, I approach the door to my building. I hobble straight to the elevator where my sister cheers me on as though I am about to cross the finish line of the New York City Marathon.

"Did you do it? Did you do it?"

I shake my head no.

"Then you can make it. You can make it. You're almost there."

We hop into the elevator and ride straight to the third floor. The pressure continues to mount in my colon. It is going to be a close one.

My sister sprints down the hallway and opens the door to my apartment. Minutes later I come around the corner. I can see the light at the end of the tunnel. My home. My bathroom.

But just as I make it to the door, the explosion starts and the warmth begins to soil my black spandex pants.

"Shit," I scream.

"No!!!"

I look at my sister and smile, *yes,* then manage to maneuver myself straight to the bathroom with no extra spillage.

I close the door behind me and quickly drop trou and let the rest out.

"I can hear that," my sister yells from the other room.

"Good. I'm glad," I say, then go back to finishing my business.

When all is said and done, I toss my pants and panties in the tub and follow them in. I turn on the shower and let the water warm as I stand to the back of the white stall.

As the cool pool at the bottom of the tub slowly clears, I make my way under the hot stream above me.

I want to cry for the pain in my knee and all that had just occurred, but all I can do is laugh.

I'd spent the last two years of my life in a state of insomnia, fearful of sleep because I worried that at any time I would wake up and not be able to walk.

Then a month ago another doctor told me I had torn the piece of cartilage between the bones of my leg and I would need surgery. When I woke from the anesthesia, I could not walk.

Every fear of the physical I'd had had came true and it wasn't even the MS that had caused the pain and paralysis. It was my own body reacting to years of running, climbing, jumping, playing soccer, and skiing. It was my enjoyment of life that had caused the surgery and the temporary loss of my ability to walk, not an invisible disease that was attacking me from the inside.

As I let the warm water of the shower fall over me, I think about how much better it is to feel pain because I'd lived, not because I'd feared the worst. Then I wonder if I'd been a fool to worry. Nights of no sleep, tears that came out of nowhere, and a deep fear that all the possible symptoms would hit me at once, are all things I had dealt with over the past 24 months. But now, they seem like they'd all been for naught. As if it were 1999 and I was like my mom preparing for the Y2K, stockpiling batteries and bottles of water for no reason. Because just like the world never fell apart and the computers never crashed, my body is still upright and strong.

Before today I was so caught up in the *what-ifs* of the unknown that I couldn't live in the present, because I was so scared of the future. What I failed to consider, however, was that while I have some sort of certainty of the future because I'd been given a list of possible symptoms and outcomes of my disease, I have no more control over my body and my future than anyone else on this planet, and I need to accept that fact.

I am not in control.

Crapping my pants at the age of 30 teaches me this lesson.

Control will never be in my reach.

I can't control my bowels. I can't control the effect the disease has on me. I can't control who loves me. And I certainly can't control who hates me, but I can finally let go and let God.

And while I may never attend an AA meeting, I now know how to surrender and accept things as they are, because...

No matter what I plan for... No matter if I worry or maintain calm... Shit is going to happen.

Chapter Twenty-Five

PUBLIC DISPLAY OF AFFECTION
(aka PDA)

My first public display of affection was on stage at the age of 13.

I had landed the part of Emily Webb in Thornton Wilder's *Our Town*. It was May of eighth grade, and it was tradition that the graduating class put on a production of a well-known play. Mr. Boetel, my English teacher and the one who taught me everything I know about sentence structure and word choice, was the director. He had cast me as the smart shy girl who finds true love with her neighbor George Gibbs, grows up, gets married, and then dies an early death.

The play was staged in a small space at Valparaiso University's student center, a ten-minute drive from my middle school. For months on end I memorized my lines and rehearsed the action. By the time opening night came around, I was ready to perform.

The first act was sweet and innocent and went along well. The romance onstage was budding and George and I were falling in love.

By the time the second act arrived we were preparing for our wedding. There were some doubts but we both proceeded on.

Backstage I dressed in a vintage wedding gown. A high neck and long sleeves covered my skin in white lace. A perfect bun was assembled atop my head before I donned a pair of heels and snuck to the back of the theatre behind the audience. When the wedding march began, my father, Mr. Webb, linked his arm in mine and pulled the veil over my eyes.

As I walked down the aisle I saw familiar faces through the haze of tulle. Jordan, the seventh grader I went to the movies with once, my choir instructor, some neighbors, Cassie and my parents, my grandparents. Step by step I inched my way to the altar, a wooden riser with a small podium placed behind it. The processional music quieted and my stage father gave me away before he walked off. The lights dimmed in the audience and a spotlight shone above George and I. We said our vows and when the priest pronounced us husband and wife, George removed the veil from my face and my lips met with his.

When we'd rehearsed the kiss at school we were supposed to "cheat it," put our faces in each other's necks and move around so it appeared that we were in love. But on that day we decided to go for it.

In front of my family, teachers, and boys whose lips had once touched my cheek, we kissed for real. My red stained lips pressed up against his and in five seconds we sealed our fate in front of everyone. The Stage Manager encouraged the crowd to clap and as we turned to them I noticed that my better half had lipstick all over his face. I panicked as I realized that if it was on his cheek then certainly it was no longer in its rightful place on my mouth. So I did what any young teenager would do, I got rid of all evidence that pointed to the fact that I had just been kissing a boy. I took the back of my hand and swiped it over my lips and face, wiping away my first brush with marriage. The audience erupted in laughter and I smiled as I interlaced my fingers with my husband's and we walked down the aisle together.

That night at home, my parents congratulated me on a performance well done, then teased me about the kiss.

"What are you going to do when you get married for real one day?" my dad asked.

"I don't know," I said. "Not wear red lipstick?"

At 13 that was my only thought on how to marry properly (or kiss in public): Keep the details of your escapades undetectable. You could kiss boys on the sidewalk, behind the bleachers, at the movies, in your parents' basement, but never let there be evidence. If he was growing scruff along his chin to prove his manhood, beware of the chafing across your cheek. If you had perfectly curled your hair, ask him to back off on the dry humping. And if you happened to get caught in the act, quickly turn it back to PG. These were the rules of PDA as a teen.

Today, in the year 2010, those rules are a little bit different for me. I can kiss him in the dark, on the kitchen table or the park, but I can never let a man learn of my affliction. For almost 36 months now, I've done my best to kiss, suck, and fuck with my face behind a veil.

I've been cheating it, fake kissing my way through all of Los Angeles.

I've resorted to being 13 again, but instead of worrying that my parents are going to discover I've been making out with a boy, I'm worried the boy's going to find out I rely on my parents for a hell of a lot more than a call at Christmas and a birthday card with cash. They are my everything when it comes to this disease. They are the ones I call in tears, who show up for appointments, and phone when they think I might be down. They are the ones who foot the bill when the MRIs clock in at thousands of dollars, and they are there when I want to fly home to escape the craziness of LA.

One month before my first MRI, I moved into a new place in Marina Del Rey.

My mom flew out to help me get settled. We unpacked boxes and rearranged furniture to take in the view. I thought the new apartment signified change, that something grand was about to happen in my life, my mom thought that "something" was the idea that the next time I moved I'd be moving in with my husband.

I was right, my mom was wrong.

Now, it is nearly three years later, and the lease on my marina apartment has run up for the third time. I contemplate my next step. I could stay and wait for my mother's prediction to come true, or I could take matters into my own hands.

I decide to do the latter and move to a new place down the street.

I make no forecasts of husbands or grand changes. I go because it is time.

On moving day, the movers come and take away all of my things and I am left alone in my old apartment.

The carpet is indented where the corners of my white couch once sat, the walls are marked by dust surrounding the space where mirrors had hung, and the kitchen is dark, full of memories of wine sipped and enjoyed.

It is the third act of the story. Emily Webb has died giving birth to her second child. She is at her funeral, then back in time at her twelfth birthday, she sees everyone from her past, but cannot linger long.

"Good-bye, good-bye, world," she says. "Good-bye, Grover's Corners… and ticking clocks…"

She continues and I join her.

"Good-bye Brad and your excuses. Good-bye Randy and the no sex rule. Good-bye Englishman, and good-bye Ryan and your miraculously cured father. Good-bye to the predictions of finding the one…"

In my now-empty apartment I am flooded with the memories of the life I've been forced to lead.

"Good-bye to the rules, and hiding the truth," I say.

I take one last look around my empty apartment. I whisper one final "good-bye," then shut the door and rotate the key, pulling the handle not once but twice to ensure it's locked forever. I turn and walk down the hallway and never return.

"Do any human beings ever realize life while they live it?" Emily asks, confounded by death.

I decide the next man I meet I will tell him upfront about the diagnosis. I don't want to cheat it anymore. I want the real thing.

I want to go out and kiss with the brightest crimson shade I can find. I want it to be messy and full of stains. I want to have to wipe my face and start over. I want the audience to laugh and I want my parents to ask me questions. I want to live in public and kiss out loud.

Part 3

Chapter Twenty-Six

STAGE FRIGHT

On a sunny February morning in 2013, I am alone on a stage.

My voice has been mic'd to carry across 50 yards, maybe further. I am on the Santa Monica Pier. Soon the Pacific Ocean will echo whispers of my words to others. For now, I am the only one here. Waves surge below and beyond. Malibu is behind me, my home in the Marina is in front. I swivel my head to take in the view of the two cities—a North/South compass to remind me where I have been and where I am now.

On the small stage I set up my yoga mat. How I got here is not easy, but can be told simply.

It took some time, but I finally found another writing job. I was hired to write a documentary on yoga. It was a different kind of writing than I was used to, but it was one that I enjoyed nonetheless. Day after day I showed up to an editing facility in Burbank, working to manifest a film that I could be proud of.

After months of sitting in a dark room, manipulating hours and hours of footage, the premiere of the film was held in Santa Monica at the Aero Theatre on Montana. I showed up that night in a new dress, a giant turquoise ring on my hand, gifted to me by my father. My name was printed boldly on the poster that hung in the showcase window at the entrance. At the end of the film, my name scrolled across the giant screen. After the screening there was a Q&A with the director. Before he took any questions he acknowledged the work of those who'd helped to create the film. I was asked to stand up in the middle of the audience. All eyes were on me.

A wave of hives brushed my neck. The red crept across my skin. But I ignored it because as the audience started to clap I realized I had accomplished everything I had ever set out to do in my professional life.

I had three goals when it came to my career: have my name in print, have my name on the small screen, and have my name on the big screen. I had never thought these things were possible and yet by the age of 31 I had done them all.

When people hear you've been diagnosed with a life-altering disease, they want you to have this big "aha" moment. This moment where you decide to do something grand with your life now that it's been altered. Maybe you buy a ticket around the world, or vow to take an oath of silence for six months, or quit your job as a salesman and become a stuntman. But the truth is, this rarely happens. And it is definitely not what happened with me. MS never gave me the desire to go out and change my life completely, it just gave me the desire to keep moving forward, however difficult that may be.

So several months after the *Titans of Yoga* documentary was released, I found myself at a new yoga studio in Venice. The owner of the studio happened to be leading a teacher training that spring. He suggested I sign up. I said I loved yoga and wanted to learn more, but there was no way I would ever teach. I hated speaking in front of people. I broke out in hives. Always.

But he was persistent and I signed up for the training. Every day for one month straight I showed up at the yoga studio and learned as much as I could about yoga and teaching. In the back of my head, I still kept saying that I would never teach, that I was just there to learn.

However, as part of our training we were required to teach a section of a one-hour class. I wrote out what I was going to say and I rehearsed it over and over, but it never came out smoothly. I felt like I was 25 again, trying to spout story ideas on cue for television producers. I thought I would fail miserably. But when I stood up that night to teach for my first time ever, the words flowed and continued to pour out my mouth and for some reason there were no hives.

I have now been teaching yoga for over two years. I have taught in various studios and exclusive gyms across LA. I have taught at corporate retreats and to small groups, but today it is different.

It is a Saturday and I have been asked to teach a class on the world-famous Santa Monica Pier. It is a big event. For the past week my photo and bio have been floating around the internet, promoted by the people who run the events at the pier. It's part of a get-healthy program. A free class for the public. A paid gig for me.

The woman who runs the event approaches and tells me we have five minutes until we start.

People begin to file in and lay down their mats. They line them up, row upon row in front of the stage I will soon inhabit. We are positioned at the very end of this historic pier, close to the tourist action but far from it all. Hundred-year-old planks of wood hold the weight of restaurants, arcades, a Ferris wheel, roller coaster, trapeze, and now, us.

I am introduced. The mic is handed over to me and my voice is loud, yet calm.

I tell the students, nearly two hundred in total, that this time is for them. That everyone is working at a different level, that as they start to flow through the poses there is no need to compare themselves to the person next to them, that their only worry should be their own body.

I take a seat on the stage and direct them to follow suit.

They sit comfortably on their mats, eyes closed. I ask them to take a deep breath in through their noses, then guide them to part their lips and exhale. The air moves in unison under the blue sky. On the next breath, I open my eyes, but instead of seeing the people in front of me, I see myself.

I am now 33 years old. Back at my apartment there is an order for two MRIs sitting on my desk—one for my spine and one for my brain. Next week I have to have those scans done and the possibility remains that this time the scans may change, but the possibility also remains that they may stay the same.

I am now on a new regimen. It's a wait and see approach.

Every six months I see the MS specialist and once a year I get brain and spinal MRIs. This will be the routine indefinitely, until something changes. If more lesions appear on my brain or my health starts to deteriorate then we will discuss another plan, like taking one of the disease modifying drugs. For now, the only drug I take is baclofen to help with the tingling and the muscle pain. Overall, my disease is at a good place, but any day that could change.

I have come to learn to live with this uncertainty. It's another facet of my life. Just like I am a girl who has a loving sister, parents, giant family; I am also a girl who teaches yoga, writes constantly, works hard, loves the outdoors, and dreams of living abroad.

I ask the students to make their way to their feet. They extend their arms to the sky. Four hundred hands reach out and beyond.

For the next hour, I give clear, concise instructions for each pose. There is no shaky voice, and no red patches on my neck.

I am at home. The words I say are all mine, the ideas I convey flow freely.

I no longer feel like the obligatory empty chair sitting in the middle of the room as the world moves around me. I am now a part of this world.

Two hundred bodies of all shapes and sizes move in synchronicity to my instructions. For the most part these people are all strangers, but there is one man I know intimately. He is in the middle of the crowd. We met online and we have been dating for several months now. Our relationship is moving slow, the way it should be. It is open and honest and there are no secrets. I smile at him across the way as the sea of bodies ebbs and flows. He smiles back and waves, then I return my focus to teaching.

When the class ends, I direct the students to make their way down onto their mats for the final resting pose. I kneel on the stage and tell the students to lie comfortably on their backs and close their eyes. I ask them to take one deep breath in, to fill up their lungs, then open their mouths and let it go. I do the same.

My exhale echoes through the speakers and resonates with theirs.

I sit in silence, taking it all in.

Six years ago I was high and alone in an MRI, now I am on a stage surrounded by hundreds. I glance up to the sky in a moment of gratitude.

After five minutes, I ask the students to slowly deepen their breath and gently wiggle their fingers and their toes. As they come back to their bodies I instruct them to make their way up to a seated position.

Once they are seated upright, I ask them to draw their hands to their hearts then gently bow their heads. I say a few words, thanking them for coming out to practice with me, then through my mic I whisper "namaste." It is a gesture of recognition that we are all in this together. That we are all on a journey, and whether that journey is epic or small, it matters.

Chapter Twenty-Seven

THE PROPOSAL

Τhe first time my dad proposed to my mom I was in utero. The second time he got on bended knee I was three glasses deep in Veuve.

It was Christmas Eve, 2010. I was visiting my parents in Chicago and my sister was in Minnesota with her boyfriend (now husband) for the holidays. My parents and I had spent the afternoon at the Four Seasons sipping champagne and feasting on roasted chicken and duck.

Our table was covered in fine white linens and our conversation bounced between memories of Christmases past and plans for the new year. We remarked about how weird it was that my sister was not there and reflected on the fact that the last time it was just the three of us I was only two.

"It's kind of like when you were younger," my dad began, "except we were probably eating mac and cheese and hot dogs 'cause that was all we could afford."

I smiled as I remembered a time when the unfurnished rooms in the house weren't left empty so that my sister and I could practice gymnastics as we believed, but were instead a reflection of their struggles to get by.

My parents were married at the age of 20 and I was born soon after. They were young and naive and I'm sure people told them they were fools to think that love was all they needed.

When I was a kid I never knew if my parents struggled or not. They shielded my sister and me from any financial talk and made sure that there was food on our plates and we enjoyed being kids.

Their song, Loggins and Messina's "Danny's Song," seemed to play throughout my childhood. The lyrics, *Even though we ain't got money, I'm so in love with you honey,* rang true for them.

As day gave way to night that Christmas Eve, we made our way back to my parents' condo. Once home my dad insisted we open another bottle of champagne and we toasted to good health and happiness. We sat in the living room and peered out the floor-to-ceiling windows as the Merchandise Mart lit up in red and green and the city lights glimmered under the blanket of white.

When my sister and I were little it was tradition that we were allowed to open one gift the night before Santa arrived. That night I chose a wrapped package that revealed itself to be an iPad. My mom, however, was not given a choice. My dad had chosen the gift for her.

He went into their room and returned with a little red leather box embossed with gold leaf. I looked at my mom and smiled. We both knew what that box meant. However, I don't think either of us expected what happened next.

My dad approached my mom on the couch and slowly lowered himself down on one knee.

"Petey," he said, as he grabbed her left hand in his.

"Gary," she exclaimed.

Tears started to form in the corners of her eyes as they did in mine.

My dad began his speech about how they had been married 30-some years and he'd always wanted to give her the ring she deserved when they first got engaged. He talked about their adventures over the years and how he was as in love with her now as he was when they first started dating. I took pictures of each moment along the way and when he said, "Will you continue to spend the rest of your life with me?" he opened the red box. My mom said, "yes," and my dad placed a band of gold and diamonds on her finger.

The last photo I took in the series is the two of them, arms wrapped around each other, my mom's ring finger shining in the light.

When they emerged from their moment, they invited me in for a family hug and I noticed that my dad was teary-eyed.

There are very few moments where I can remember my dad crying, the last being when my parents renewed their vows in Vegas for their 25th wedding anniversary. My sister and I went along as maids of honor and stood as witnesses as they promised again to love each other eternally. Our family of four laughed and cried and my sister and I fought over the bouquet, hoping to be next.

It takes a certain kind of love to make a marriage work. I know about this love in the same way I know what it means to work hard and get what you want in this world, because I've lived with a perfect example of it since the cells of my body were barely beginning to form. It's a love that is infinite and unconditional. My parents aren't saints and I'm sure they've had plenty of ups and downs in their lives, but the overwhelming message I've received from them throughout my entire life is that love conquers all.

Through every bended knee my dad got down on, and every walk down the aisle my parents took together, I have been there. If that's not proof that everlasting love is possible then I don't know what is.

What I do know, however, is that it's their love that's showed me why the MS has affected me so deeply.

On that fateful October day years ago I cried to my dad, "Who's going to want to marry me now?" At the time, I didn't know where that thought came from, but I said it and I believed it.

Today, I believe it came from my innate understanding of unconditional love and my idea that it would be challenging to develop that kind of love with a man knowing that being with me came with many conditions.

I believed loving me was like loving a ticking time bomb. That I had a clock that would inevitably expire and no matter how many red or blue wires were cut or disconnected, something would eventually explode and someone would have to clean up the mess. The possibility of paralysis, incontinence, trips to the ER, constant pain, lack of sex drive, depression—these were all things anyone who chose to be with me might one day have to learn to love.

When I was little I asked my dad, "How do you know when you're supposed to marry someone?"

"You'll just know," he said.

When my sister married in 2013, I was the maid of honor. I got up in front of nearly 175 people and gave my speech. I talked about my sister and her husband and their love for each other, but when I got to the part where I was to make a toast this is what I said:

"There is one person who is not here today and I wish she were. My Grandma Reed passed away years ago, but I still remember her fondly. She was a little quirky and was known for saying random things. When things weren't looking so good for any of us, she'd always say, 'Don't worry, you come from good stock.' When I was young I thought,

Great, I'm super strong and I'll be healthy forever. But now that I'm older I have a new interpretation. And that is, that coming from good stock means we come from a lot of love. But it's not just that we know how to love, it's that we're very good at surrounding ourselves with those who know what it means to love unconditionally. So let's all raise our glasses and cheers to the fact that by choosing each other, Cassie and Taylor have brought together a room full of people who come from good stock."

After my speech I hugged my sister and new brother-in-law and returned to my seat. To the left of me were my cousin and her husband and to my right was my date, the man I had met online. At that point he had been in my life for nearly nine months. When I'd told him about the MS we were at dinner on one of our first dates. He asked a few questions about how I was doing and I responded that I was actually doing quite well. Half an hour later when I returned from a trip to the ladies' room, I discovered that he had spent the last five minutes looking up the disease, educating himself. He said nothing except that there was hope and he was willing to look for it with me.

I have always wanted what my parents have, a love that cannot be explained, just understood.

Throughout our house growing up there were pictures and paintings and statues of birds. Why? I don't know. But it was something my parents held on to as a secret symbol of their love. It's part of the mystery of why it works for them and I will never know, but that is okay, because it is their story and one day I will have my own.

As the night of my sister's wedding went on, I watched as my date mingled with my family. My grandpa told him stories of me as a child, my aunts surrounded him on the dance floor, my parents bombarded him with questions. But through it all he kept a smile on his face.

It would be another three months before he said, "I love you," and another 13 before we moved in together, but it would be well worth the wait. How do I know this? I just know.

Acknowledgements

I remember the day I decided to write this book quite vividly. I was sitting in the waiting room at the lab at UCLA getting ready to have blood drawn. I had just seen the specialist and she had reiterated what the neurologist had said: I believe you have multiple sclerosis. My parents were sitting with me and the three of us were pretty silent. The reality of what the specialist had said was settling into our lives. My mind was racing. Suddenly, I turned to my parents and said, "I have an idea." I pitched them the story about incontinence and my fear of pissing my pants and trying to date through it all. They laughed and said, "You should write that book." Since that day they have never stopped supporting every idea I ever had. They have read countless iterations of this memoir and listened to me complain about all the frogs I kissed along the way. They have accompanied me to more doctor appointments than I care to remember and they have footed the medical bills when I could no longer afford to pay them on my own. To say I am a lucky daughter is an understatement. Mom and Dad thank you for being my rock, yesterday, today and forever more. I love you from here to eternity.

To my baby sister, Cassie, thank you for being the comic relief to the roller coaster that has been the last nine years. You are my best friend, and my confidante. You push me out of my comfort zone and keep me in check. I promise, if you ever find yourself nearing the edge of shitting your pants I will run ahead and open all the doors for you. Because, as you've shown me, that's what sisterly love is all about and I love you dearly.

To my extended family, Grandma and Papa, my mass amount of aunts and uncles and my gazillion cousins, thank you for your kind words along the way—the conversations, the emails, the pats on the back. Facing illness is never easy, but knowing you have an army to back you up is the most comforting thing a girl could ask for.

Thank you to my friends, Colleen, Brooke, Emily, Misty, Robin, Tyler, Becky, Stephanie and Jen. You girls have been there since day one of this journey. While I may have kept quiet about much of what I've gone through, you have always been there to support me. Your friendships are invaluable.

I have loved writing since I was a young girl, but I would not be where I am today if it weren't for the incredible teachers I've had along the way. To my seventh and eighth grade English teacher, Mr. Boetel, thank you for teaching me everything I know. You are the foundation to all I have ever written. To my high school teachers Mr. Bird and Mrs. Watson, thank you for encouraging my creativity. And to my college professors, David St. John, T.C. Boyle and Aimee Bender, thank you for being prime examples of what it means to be a professional writer. You solidified my desire to make writing my career.

I feel blessed to have a circle of friends who are all writers in their own right. They've helped me find my voice and pushed me to continue writing when I wanted to give up. To Cormac and Marianne Wibberley thank you for reading various versions of this book and always being willing to help in any way you could. Your support has been a godsend. To Joyce Actor and the amazing group of writers you put together—Jim, Gerry, James, Kate, Gloria and Susan— if it weren't for the incredible feedback you all gave me I might still be writing this book. To Deanne Stillman and the writers of the UCLA writing class I attended just one month after I was diagnosed, thank you for planting the seeds to this memoir.

To my editor Emily Heckman, thank you for your honesty. You pushed me to expand my story and turn it into something great. To my other editor Deri Reed, thank you for getting me as a writer. You understood my voice and made sure it shined clear.

To all of my doctors, thank you for treating me like a person and not just a patient. If I have learned anything from this experience, it is that not all doctors are created equal. Thank you for being my support team for good health.

To all those living with MS who have shared their stories online or in person, thank you for being so open and honest and making a girl feel less alone. I can only hope that I can do the same for others one day.

Last but not least, thank you Greg for showing me that I am still lovable. It is your love that has pushed me to the final step of publishing this book. Without you I might still be afraid, but with you by my side I have the confidence to go out and share my story with others. I love you.

CPSIA information can be obtained at www.ICGtesting.com
Printed in the USA
LVOW11*1222050716

495027LV00001B/1/P